MAIMONIDES &METABOLISM

MAIMONIDES &METABOLISM

Physiology of Fat-Loss

**Maimonides Method of Diet and Exercise
For Curing the Metabolic Syndrome:
Obesity, Type 2 Diabetes, and Heart Disease**

A presentation of his most relevant teachings concerning diet
and exercise, explained in the light of the most cutting-edge
research in physiology and endocrinology

Rabbi Yonason Herschlag

ISBN: 0692651683
ISBN-13: 9780692651681
Library of Congress Control Number: 2015904595
CreateSpace Independent Publishing Platform
North Charleston, South Carolina
Distributed by INGRAM
Website: idealmetabolism.com
Author email: herschlag@012.net.il or yonasonherschlag@gmail.com

Table of Contents

Preface ·xi

Introduction · xv

**Part I: The Paradox: How Restricting Calories Makes
Some People Fatter** · 1

Chapter 1   Fat Mass Is Dependent on Hormonal Balance · · · · · · · · · · · 3

Chapter 2   How to Decrease Your Fat Cell Number · · · · · · · · · · · · · · 17

Chapter 3   Customizing Your Fat-Mass Reduction Plan · · · · · · · · · · 25

Part II: The Metabolic Syndrome
Obesity, Prediabetes, and Heart Disease: Developing
Lifelong Habits for Better Health and Insulin Sensitivity · 33

Chapter 4   The Metabolic Syndrome: Its Causes and Remedies · · · · · 35

Chapter 5   Benefits of an Early Dinner · 47

Chapter 6   Exercise: The Benefits, How and When,
and Making It Easy · 53

Chapter 7   Late Breakfast: When, Why, and What to Eat · · · · · · · · · · 75

Appendix to
Chapter 7   Late Breakfast: The Moral Significance According to
the Talmud · 85

Chapter 8   Measured Glycemic Load: Avoiding Hyperinsulinemia · · · 89

Chapter 9   Daily Intermittent Fasting · 97

Part III: Macronutrients

What the Body Uses Them for, Recommended
Sources, How Much We Need, and Planning a Healthy
and Balanced Diet· 107

Chapter 10 RDA of Macronutrients (Carbohydrates,
Proteins, and Fats) · 109

Chapter 11 Protein· 121

Chapter 12 Carbohydrates: Sugar, Starch, and Fiber · · · · · · · · · · · · 135

Appendix to
Chapter 12: The Different Structure and Different Physiological
Effects of Sugars, Starches, and Fiber · · · · · · · · · · · · · · · 153

Chapter 13 Fats · 157

Appendix to
Chapter 13: Understanding the Terms *Saturated, Unsaturated,
Polyunsaturated, Cis,* and *Trans* · · · · · · · · · · · · · · · · · · · 177

Part IV: Comparative Study of Popular Diets

An Examination of Many Studies Determining
the Most Effective Methods for Weight Loss and
Improvement of Metabolic Parameters · · · · · · · · · · · · · · 181

Chapter 14 Benefits of Low-Carbohydrate Diets· · · · · · · · · · · · · · · 183

Chapter 15 Pros and Cons of Some of the Most Popular Diets· · · · · · 213

Chapter 16 Combining the Most Effective Methods for Short-Term
and Long-Term Fat Loss · 257

Glossary · 277

Bibliography · 285

About the Author · 319

Disclaimer:

The information provided herein is a resource for personal study; it does not constitute medical or diet advice (which needs to be customized according to one's individual needs). Consult a doctor or licensed dietitian before making significant diet changes.

If you find some information here to be incorrect or misleading, I encourage you to inform me, and if there is sufficient evidence to demonstrate the need for a correction, I will happily post that on my website, idealmetabolism.com, and incorporate that into the next edition.

One of my favorite hobbies is home improvement. With a pick and shovel, I dug the foundations to add two rooms to our house; bent and formed the rebar for the pillars and beams; built stone-faced reinforced cement walls from scratch; installed the electric and plumbing for the new kitchen, bathroom, and office; installed the floor tiling; and more—virtually completing the entire project with my own hands. For the ceiling, I needed an additional pair of hands to set up the temporary support beams in preparation for pouring the cement, so my wife assisted with that.

When my wife was in the hospital for the delivery of our seventh child eight years ago, I decided to surprise her with some more new improvements to welcome her home. What a surprise she got! While climbing out of a window, I twisted my knee, tore the meniscus, and couldn't even pick myself up off the floor. Eventually I was carted off to the hospital for surgery.

Prior to this knee injury at age forty-four, I had been running daily and lifting weights occasionally. However, recovery from the knee surgery was quite slow; it was only after three years that I regained full flexibility. By that time I had gained a lot of weight, even though I ate sensibly, exercised, went to dietitians, and made numerous attempts at weight loss. A combination of a variety of stresses and the hormonal changes associated with middle age simply frustrated every effort I made to lose weight. Despite my being quite disciplined, my waistline continued its expanding trend.

When I was twenty-two years old and suffered a ruptured disc in an auto collision, I swam my way to recovery, eventually becoming a certified lifeguard and swimming instructor. At age forty-nine, with a forty-four-inch waist and the realization that calorie restriction wouldn't work for me, I decided to once again exercise my way to good health, but there was no gym in my city. So I built one.

Running the gym wouldn't have been practical without becoming a licensed trainer, so I joined the program at the prestigious Wingate Institute in Jerusalem. It was there that I began learning physiology, but the more I learned, the more fascinated and the more driven I became to have an even greater understanding. I then accumulated a library of diet and exercise books and medical textbooks and utilized Google to discover many important studies.

Beyond some bare basics in becoming certified as a fitness trainer, I never had a formal education in physiology. After studying on my own and taking notes, I assumed that I could present the physiology of fat loss in a simple layperson's language. But the reality is that the way the body works is very complex. So even though I present the physiology of fat loss as simply as I can, it still takes much dedication to the subject to digest all these ideas.

My experience tells me that books on health written by people with a background primarily in the Talmud are full of misinformation, despite the sincere good intentions. With my scanty formal scientific background, I was afraid I was in the same boat. But I was pleasantly surprised when health professionals (dietitians, doctors, etc.) expressed their amazement at how much they learned from my book. Additionally, several health professionals have told me how they really enjoyed the ease of grasping new and complex ideas as presented here.

My credentials are not that I did eight reps of a 484-pound deadlift less than seven weeks after my second knee surgery at age fifty-two (you can see the video on our website idealmetabolism.com), nor the fact that after twenty years working as a religious scribe and many failed attempts at reducing weight through a variety of conventional and non-conventional methods, I discovered a combination of techniques to get my waistline down from forty-four inches to thirty-eight. Nor are my credentials a certificate or degree. Rather my credentials are the value of the contents of this book, which are recognized and appreciated by a growing number of health professionals.

There are two things that enabled me to bring a fresh perspective and "new" methods into the scientific world:

1. my application of the teachings of the Talmud and Maimonides to the world of physiology, and
2. an unusual talent for thorough and in-depth research.

Millions of people have been frustrated with standard dieting techniques promoted by the "authorities." Many people are stricken with a metabolism that makes it impossible to succeed with conventional diet techniques, myself included. When I use the word *metabolism*, I am referring to the chemical transformations that take place inside our cells, both catabolism and anabolism. A simplified explanation of these terms is that *catabolism* is the process of breaking down chemical structures, usually for the purpose of harnessing life-sustaining energy from them, and *anabolism* is the process of building biochemical structures for a broad array of functions that the body needs to maintain life.

Most people would like to see their anabolic processes build their muscle and keep their bodies strong and vibrant, while their catabolic processes break down and burn off their excess body fat. However, the frustration of many people (especially those middle aged and beyond) is that their genetic predisposition combined with the influences of life does just the reverse of our desires; the catabolic processes diminish our body's lean mass, while our anabolic processes are focused on building up more and more body fat, as though our bodies were preparing for a famine of biblical proportions.

The metabolic directions inside of us are regulated by the hypo-thalamus, a small part of the brain located at its base. The hypothalamus controls body temperature, hunger, thirst, fatigue, sleep, and more. It's somewhat infantile to teach that consuming five hundred calories fewer per day will knock off one pound of fat per week. If your hypothalamus wants to store fat, it can manage that—even if you cut your calories from three thousand per day down to fifteen hundred per day—by using energy more efficiently. And if your hypothalamus decides to burn fat, you can eat more while absorbing less, and your hypothalamus can direct your metabolism to burn loads of fat, just like you can burn off gas and electric fuel by turning on the air conditioning and heating at the same time.

So the question is, how can we influence our hypothalamus to direct metabolism according to our desires? That's what *Maimonides and Metabolism* is about.

Introduction

M *aimonides and Metabolism* is not a translation of the numerous, lengthy, and complex medical works of Maimonides but rather a new presentation of select health principles that are found in Maimonides's writings. The focus is on the relevance of Maimonides's diet and exercise principles to some of the primary health concerns of our time (predominantly the metabolic syndrome—obesity, diabetes, and heart disease) and understanding his recommendations within the context of the most up-to-date principals of physiology and endocrinology.

Concerning diet, the focus of the past few decades has been on *what* foods to avoid and include. More recently there has been a shift in focus on *when* to eat and *how often* to eat. There were widespread recommendations to eat more often, and more recently, intermittent fasting has become popular. Many dietitians stress the importance of not skipping breakfast, but this is far from a clear-cut issue and is now a topic of hot debate. Similarly there are those who recommend a prebedtime snack and those who argue against it.

In part II: chapters 4 through 9, I explain and expound on the benefits of gradually adapting to Maimonides's recommendations of

1. avoiding late-night snacks,
2. pushing off breakfast until at least three hours after awakening, and
3. doing aerobic exercise before meals (especially breakfast).

And these chapters are solidly backed up with explanations based on the most up-to-date physiology and endocrinology theory and studies.

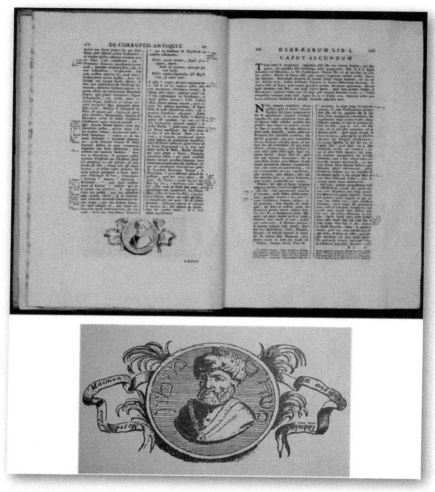

Figure I-1. Rabbi Isacco Samuele Reggio (b. 1784–d. 1855) located this portrait of Maimonides in a thirty-four-volume encyclopedic work called *Thesaurus Antiquitatum Sacrarum*, which was published between 1744 and 1769 by Blaseus Ugolinus in Venice. Written in Latin, it is a thesaurus of sacred antiquities that illustrates the customs and laws of sacred and civil rights of the ancient Hebrews.

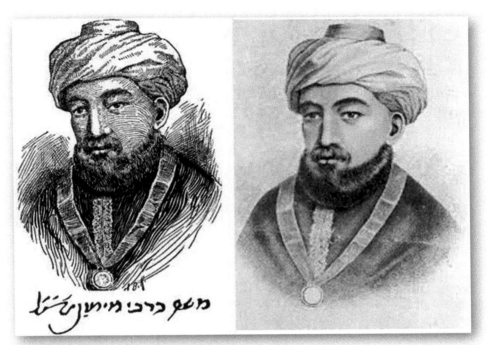

Figure I-2. Left—ink portrait of Maimonides with signature by an unknown artist. Right—later pastel rendition. Based on figure I-1, an unknown artist made this ink drawing (figure I-2, left), adding a copy of Maimonides's signature. More recently, a different unknown artist converted the above ink drawing into the famous pastel rendition (figure I-2, right).

MAIMONIDES: A PARTIAL BIOGRAPHY

Rabbi Moshe ben Maimon, also known as Rambam and commonly known as Maimonides, was a Talmudist, codifier of Jewish law, physician, philosopher, and communal leader. He is the most famous Jewish doctor of all time; many hospitals and schools across the globe are named after him.

In his ancient medical writings, Maimonides described many conditions, including asthma, diabetes, hepatitis, and pneumonia. He emphasized moderation and a healthy lifestyle. His treatises became influential for generations of physicians. He was knowledgeable about Greek and Arabic medicine and the principles of humoral medicine in the tradition of Galen.[1] He did not blindly accept the medical theories of his era but rather used his own observation and experience combined with his extensive knowledge of anatomy and medicine based on traditional Torah sources in his application of contemporary medical wisdoms.

From Spain to Egypt

Moshe Maimonides was born in Cordoba, Spain, on the eve of Passover in 1135 CE, nearly nine hundred years ago. His father, Maimon, a direct descendant of King David, was a judge in the city's rabbinical court.[2]

The word for *son* in Hebrew is "ben." As such, Moshe, the son of Maimon, was known as Rabbi Moshe Ben Maimon (Rabbi Moshe, the son of Maimon). His Hebrew acronym is the English equivalent of *RMBM*, pronounced Rambam; thus, in Hebrew literature, he is most commonly referred to as "the Rambam."

When Maimonides was thirteen, his family was forced to flee Cordoba when a fanatic Islamic sect took control of the city. Not finding anything suitable in Spain, he and his father and younger brother, David, moved to Fez, Morocco, for five years. At age thirty, he visited the land of Israel and then moved to Alexandria, Egypt. Later, he settled in Fustat—today known as Old Cairo—where he lived until his passing at age sixty-nine.[3]

In Egypt, Maimonides was supported by his brother David, a merchant who imported diamonds from India. His brother's financial support gave Maimonides the ability to devote himself to the study of the Torah and to author his scholarly works.

However, in 1171, when Maimonides was thirty-six, his brother David drowned when his ship sunk en route to India. Without any

---

1 Fred Rosner, "The Life of Moses Maimonides: Prominent Medieval Physician," *Einstein Quartet Journal of Biology and Medicine* (2002): 125–28, https://www.einstein.yu.edu/uploadedFiles/EJBM/19Rosner125.pdf.

2 Dovid Zaklikowski, *Maimonides: His Life and Works*. See also www.chabad.org.

3 Zaklikowski, *Maimonides*.

further support from his brother, Maimonides began practicing medicine in an effort to support himself and his brother's family.[4]

Maimonides the Doctor

In his midfifties, Maimonides was appointed as a personal physician to Saladin, the king of Egypt and Syria.

Maimonides composed works of Jewish scholarship, rabbinic law, philosophy, and medical texts. He also wrote ten known medical works in Arabic:[5]

- *Extracts from Galen*, or *The Art of Cure*: an extract of Galen's extensive writings
- *Commentary on the Aphorisms of Hippocrates*: A text interspersed with Maimonides's own views
- *Medical Aphorisms of Moses* (*Fusul Musa* in Arabic and *Pirkei Moshe* [Chapters of Moses] in Hebrew): fifteen hundred aphorisms, in which many medical conditions are described
- *Treatise on Hemorrhoids*: discusses digestion and food
- *Treatise on Cohabitation*: contains recipes as aphrodisiacs and anti-aphrodisiacs
- *Treatise on Asthma*: discusses climates and diets and their effect on asthma, and emphasizes the need for clean air
- *Treatise on Poisons and Their Antidotes*: an early toxicology textbook that remained popular for centuries
- *Regimen of Health*: a discourse on healthy living and the mind-body connection
- *Discourse on the Explanation of Fitness*: advocates healthy living and the avoidance of overindulgence

---

4 Ibid.
5 Fred Rosner, "The Life of Moses Maimonides,": Prominent Medieval Physician," *Einstein Quartet Journal of Biology and Medicine* (2002): 125–28, https://www.einstein. yu.edu/uploadedFiles/EJBM/19Rosner125.pdf.

- *Glossary of Drug Names*: represents a pharmacopeia with 405 paragraphs with the names of drugs in Arabic, Greek, Syrian, Persian, Berber, and Spanish

In addition to these ten medical works, Maimonides's famous code of Jewish law, *Mishneh Torah*, also includes a small section dedicated to prescriptions for health, including basic principles of diet, exercise, and emotional and physical health.

Even with the knowledge that Saladin, the King of Egypt and Syria, considered him the greatest doctor of the generation and that his writings on medicine and health were considered essential texts for generations, it is still impossible to recognize the greatness of Maimonides's knowledge of medicine and how far ahead of his time he was without an awareness of how outstanding his knowledge of Jewish law was.

Maimonides: The Greatest Codifier of Jewish Law

Despite having sacrificed so much of his time to healing the sick, Maimonides became one of the most important figures in the history of Torah scholarship. On his gravestone in Tiberias, Israel, is inscribed, "From Moshe to Moshe, none arose as Moshe." This suggests that from the biblical Moshe, who led the Jewish people out of slavery in Egypt and gave us the Pentateuch, up until Moshe Maimonides, who gave us the Mishneh torah, there was no teacher of Jewish law as outstanding as they.

Maimonides wrote numerous books on Judaism. His most monumental and historically outstanding work is his codification of Jewish law, called *Mishneh Torah*, or "Repetition of the Torah." The fourteen-volume work is a logical systematic codification of Jewish law. Figure I-3 shows the inner cover of the 1574 edition of the *Mishneh Torah*.

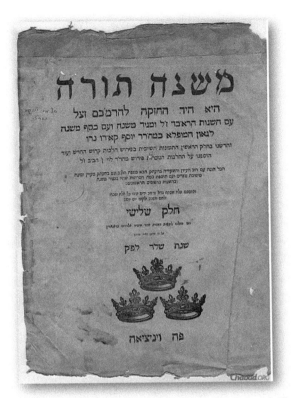

Figure I-3. Inner cover of the Rambam's Mishneh Torah
from the 1574 edition printed in Venice, Italy

Prior to Maimonides, in order to know Jewish law, one had to learn the entire Talmud. The Talmud is not merely a compilation of Jewish law but more importantly a method and practice of Jewish thinking, analyzing, and reasoning—the study of which was designed to form a person's mind and soul for divine service. It is not merely a collection of informative teachings but a larger guide for the traditional teacher-student relationship. As such, the Talmud often quotes conflicting opinions on a specific Jewish law to provoke the student of Talmud to think deeply and determine on his own which opinion is the final law.

The difficulty was that the Talmudic rulings, as well as the commentaries, were not organized in a strictly encyclopedic, orderly fashion. For example, in order to study the laws of Shabbat by exploring the Talmud, one needed to search and sift through many tractates. As such, obtaining knowledge of Jewish law required extremely taxing research, time, and dedication—something that only full-time rabbinic scholars could achieve, leaving the working masses sadly distant from its acquisition.[6]

Maimonides was the first one to index the entire body of ancient Jewish traditional teachings. And he compiled it all in a logical and systematic fashion. For example, he gathered the laws of Shabbat—which were spread out and dispersed throughout numerous tractates of Talmud—in the third volume of the Mishneh Torah in thirty chapters, dividing each into bite-sized subsections. This volume, which he titled *Zmanim*, or *Times*, contains all laws pertaining to Shabbat and holidays.

Maimonides codified laws of Shabbat, holidays, prayer, dietary laws, and the laws that regulate the Jew's daily life. The Mishneh Torah also incorporates the basics of Jewish thought and belief. He also wrote a section on eating healthy, fitness, and mental health—teaching that all our actions should be permeated with holiness and godliness. His teachings include the principle that maintaining the health and well-being of the body is part of one's religious duty.

As far as Jewish law, Maimonides was more than a trailblazer; to this very day, the Mishneh Torah remains the only work of this scope. No other work—authored beforehand or afterward—covers the entire corpus of Jewish law.[7] Maimonides not only organized and simplified Jewish law, making it so much more accessible, but he did so in a language style and with a clarity understandable to all Jews, —scholars and laymen alike.

---

6 Zaklikowski, *Maimonides: His Life and Works.* . See also www.chabad.org.
7 Ibid.

MAIMONIDES ENCODED IN THE BIBLE

To appreciate this coding, you need to understand the Jewish signifi-cance of the numbers 613 and fifty. According to the Kabbalistic tradi-tion, G-d created the human soul with 613 parts, which are divided into two categories—365 "negative" and 248 "positive." The human soul is reflected in the human body, which is also comprised anatomically of 365 categories of tendons (there are actually over four thousand ten-dons in the human body) and 248 limbs. The Talmud relates that there are 613 biblical commandments, divided into two categories: 365 *pro-hibitions* and 248 *positive commandments*. Some examples of prohibitions would be to not to worship other gods, to not steal or murder, to not eat *treifa* animals, to not eat meat cooked in its mother's milk, to not slander or lie, and so forth. Some examples of positive commandments would be to eat matzoh on the night of Passover, to recite specific vers-es of the Torah every morning and night, to love one's friend as oneself, to build a sanctuary through which to serve G-d, and so on. According to kabbalah, the observance of these 613 commandments nourishes the 613 spiritual limbs and tendons of the human. In brief, the number 613 represents something utterly essential to the human creation and the teachings of the Torah.

Another important number in the Torah is fifty. Many verses of the Torah speak about seven times seven followed by the number fifty, such as the jubilee year. Fifty days after the Exodus from Egypt, the Jewish people stood at Mount Sinai and received the Torah! There is actually a biblical commandment to count seven weeks of seven days to con-nect the two festivals—Passover and Shavuot (Shavuot literally means "weeks"). Shavuot is the festival commemorating the receiving of the Torah fifty days after the Exodus.

Keep in mind what was mentioned previously—that Rabbi Moshe Ben Maimon, more commonly referred to as the RaMBaM is in Jewish history the most *marvelous* teacher of Judaism since biblical Moshe, the son of Amram.

If we were to search where the Rambam's name and the name of his historic work, Mishneh Torah, are hidden (encoded) in the Torah, it would make the most sense to search around the verse Exodus 11:9: "And G-d spoke to Moshe, 'Pharaoh will not heed you, in order to increase My marvels in the land of Egypt.'" This verse is an obvious place to search for hints to Rabbi Moshe Ben Maimon, because since the ten marvelous plagues of the Exodus from Egypt, the Rambam and his historic teachings are the greatest *marvels* that came out of *Egypt*.

If we begin from the Hebrew letter *mem* in the first letter of the word "Moshe" in this verse and count fifty letters, we arrive at the letter *shin*. Continuing another fifty letters, we arrive at the letter *nun*. With another fifty letters, we arrive at *heh*. *Mem-shin-nun-heh* spell the Hebrew word *Mishneh*. If we then skip 613 letters, we arrive at the letter *tof*. Proceeding to count another fifty letters, we arrive at the letter *vov*. Another fifty letters brings us to the letter *resh*. Another fifty letters brings us to *heh*. *Tof-vov-resh-heh* spell the Hebrew word *Torah*.

In short, the words *Mishneh Torah* are encoded in this chapter via intervals of fifty letters between one letter and the next, with an interval of 613 letters between the word *Mishneh* and the word *Torah*!

Now let's take a closer look at the words of this verse: "Increase My marvels in the land of Egypt." In Hebrew, this is expressed in four words: *rabos* ("increase"), *mofsy* ("my marvels"), *b-eretz* ("in the land of"), and *Mitzrayim* ("Egypt"). The initial letters of these four words spell out the acrostic Rambam—**R**abbi **M**oshe **B**en **M**aimon—G-d's increase of marvel in the land of Egypt is certainly the Rambam.

ANCIENT JEWISH WISDOM

One example of amazing ancient Jewish wisdom is the Talmudic teaching that a lunar cycle is twenty-nine days, twelve hours, and 793/1080 parts of an hour.[8] In other words, a lunar cycle is 29.53059 days, exactly the same approximation as made by NASA.

---

8 Rabban Gamliel, *Tractate Rosh HaShona*, 25.

Another example revolves around a biblical injunction regarding the prohibition of eating animals that were sick or injured before being slaughtered: "Be holy to me, do not eat the flesh of a *treifa* in the field, rather throw it to the dogs" (Ex 22:30). In this context, the Hebrew word *treifa* means a torn animal (most commonly torn by wild beasts). Jewish tradition teaches that this commandment also forbids eating the flesh of animals that had such an injury or disease that would have prevented the animal from surviving more than a year. Some injuries could be obvious; for example, if a wild bull was hunted and shot down with an arrow that pierced its lungs—even if it was still breathing, even if it was standing on its feet, even if the hunter performed the Jewish ritual slaughter—the animal would not be considered permissible to eat because before the ritual slaughter, the animal suffered an injury that it could not have survived long with, therefore rendering it a *treifa*. However, there are many other injuries and diseases for which it would be difficult even for top veterinarians in our advanced, modern age to determine whether it is survivable for more than a year.

In the Mishneh Torah, Maimonides enumerates *seventy* diseases and injuries that render an animal *treifa!*[9] Maimonides's source of this magnificent wisdom is primarily the Talmud. The Talmud recorded the oral traditions concerning this wisdom handed down from teacher to student traced back to the biblical Moses. This is an astounding example of the ancient Jewish wisdom concerning physiology.

CONCLUSION

Maimonides was one of the greatest Jewish sages of all time and wrote extensively on matters of health. This book is my humble presentation of his most relevant teachings concerning diet and exercise and an attempt to explain those teachings in the light of the most advanced science of physiology and endocrinology.

---

9 Maimonides, *Mishneh Torah*, Kedusha (the book of Holiness), hilchot machlot issurot (laws of forbidden foods), chapter 4.

The book is divided into four parts. Part I deals with the paradox of how reducing calories can actually increase fat cell number, and it includes techniques for reducing fat cell number and attaining long-term fat loss. Part II is the section that delves into Maimonides's recommendations (early dinner, late breakfast, and exercise before meals) and the long-term health benefits of these recommendations (improving insulin sensitivity and curing the metabolic syndrome). Part III goes in depth into macronutrients, enabling laymen and health professionals alike to learn the best combinations of macronutrients for short- and long-term goals such as fat loss and muscle building. And part IV examines the pros and cons of a host of popular diets, concluding with the best combinations of techniques for both short- and long-term dieting.

It should be noted that while this book delves in deeply into the physiological benefits of Maimonides's recommendations concerning early dinner, late breakfast, and exercise before meals, Maimonides has some additional recommendations that I do not expand upon in this book. He writes:

1. Don't eat unless you are hungry.
2. Don't drink unless you are thirsty.
3. Don't stuff yourself full with each meal, but rather only eat until you feel three-quarters full.
4. Don't engage in excessive body movement or exertion after eating a meal until after the food is well digested (roughly one and a half or two hours).
5. Constipation can cause much harm and should be avoided by eating foods that keep the bowels loose. (In circumstances in which one needs a powerful flush—for example after a day of festive meals, or when constipated—a glass of prune juice at least a half an hour before breakfast, followed by a citrus fruit works fast to clear the intestinal tract, and detoxifies the body

quite well. However, on a day to day basis, following a high-fiber diet plan is the healthiest way to maintain loose bowels).

Maimonides also gives amazing advice about maintaining emotional health and teaches general principles on taking care of our souls. Physical health is directly affected by spiritual and emotional health; I touch upon this briefly in the appendix to chapter 7, as the Talmud connects a moral significance to delaying breakfast. However, except for that appendix, what I have compiled here focuses just on the *physiology* of fat loss through diet and exercise, primarily material that adds some new beneficial knowledge to those that have already cultivated an interest in this subject.

Part I
The Paradox: How Restricting Calories Makes Some People Fatter

Fat Mass Is Dependent on Hormonal Balance

INTRODUCTION

While the concept of weight loss via calorie restriction is not integral to Maimonides's teachings, this book would not be complete without addressing this widely misunderstood and crucial subject. Therefore, I have dedicated the first part of this book to explain how restricting calories makes some people fatter.

Maimonides's diet recommendations have a *direct* impact on improving insulin sensitivity and stabilizing blood sugar and only an *indirect* effect on fat reduction. However, since most people who struggle to lose weight commonly regain the weight they lost, it is imperative for the dieter to know why restricting calories makes some people fatter and how to avoid that weight gain.

Many doctors promote the idea that obesity is a result of self-indulgence and lack of self-discipline.[10] These doctors are supported by mainstream health authorities who promote weight-loss strategy as simple mathematics of digesting fewer calories than you burn: "A

---

10 A prime example is Dr. Pierre Dukan in the most popular diet book of all time, *The Dukan Diet* (New York: Crown Archetype, 2011), in which he says, "Not by accident are fat individuals overweight; their gourmet appetite, gluttony, and apparent lack of restraint conceals a need to find comfort in food" and "An overweight person will admit that they are weak and even immature" (1–2).

calorie is a calorie. To create weight loss, you must change the balance in favor of calories out."[11]

This misinformation is harmful, both because it leads some people to gain weight and because it mistakenly leads dieters to think they are at fault, guilty, and failures at dieting. Not only have many health authorities failed to give helpful advice, but some of their advice has actually contributed to the growing prevalence of obesity and diabetes.

FAT MASS IS DEPENDENT ON HORMONAL BALANCE

To understand the paradox of calorie restriction leading to weight gain, we need to understand the biomechanics of four particular hormones: insulin, cortisol, ghrelin, and leptin.

As hormonal balance is so integral to the physiology of fat loss, and as discussion of hormones is a central focus of this book, it is necessary that we begin by first precisely defining the word *hormone* as is relevant to our subject:

"A chemical produced by living cells (usually a combination of amino acids forming a unique structure) that circulate in body fluids (primarily blood), and that trigger specific physiological reactions when contacting the receptor of other cells (often remote from its point of origin)."

The following is a simplified abbreviated explanation of these four hormones, what part of the body primarily produces them, what triggers their production and release, and how they affect our bodies.

Insulin

Produced in the pancreas and released when blood sugar levels are too high, this hormone speeds up the absorption of nutrients, primarily in muscle tissue and the liver, thereby lowering blood sugar levels by transferring

---

11 American Heart Association, *The No-Fad Diet* (2011), 13. The book is written by a staff of half a dozen doctors and professors, with an additional dozen experts serving as advisors.

sugar out of the blood and into the muscles and liver. It also triggers the liver to convert excess sugar into fat, which then gets taken up by fat tissues.

Cortisol

Produced in the adrenal cortex and released in reaction to stress and/ or when blood sugar levels are too low, this hormone triggers the liver to release stored fat and sugar into the blood. When glycogen (stored sugar) supplies are low in the liver, cortisol directs the liver to convert fats and proteins into sugar to further contribute to raising blood sugar levels. While affected slightly by stress and blood sugar levels, cortisol blood levels are dictated primarily by a circadian rhythm (figure 1-1), which typically reaches a low point around midnight and thereafter at 2:00 a.m. begins a steep climb upward until reaching its pinnacle at 8:30 a.m. (for a person who wakes up at 8:00 a.m.). Levels then turn downward until midnight, with one to three slight rises upward over the course of the day (most notably at midday). Peak cortisol blood concentration after waking up is about eight times the concentration of the daily low point.[12]

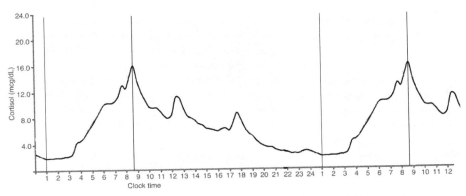

Figure 1-1. Fluctuations in Cortisol level around the clock

---

12   Sharon Chan and Miguel Debono, "Replication of Cortisol Circadian Rhythm: New Advances in Hydrocortisone Replacement Therapy," *Therapeutic Advances in Endocrinology and Metabolism* (June 2010), http://www.ncbi.nlm.nih.gov/pmc/articles/PMC3475279/.

Ghrelin

This hormone is produced in the stomach and released just prior to habituated meal times. Ghrelin increases appetite via receptors in the hypothalamus and directs metabolism to store fat as opposed to burn it, and it increases the number of fat cells via receptors in fat cells by inducing the proliferation and differentiation of adipocytes (fat cells) and inhibiting apoptosis (programed cell death/self-destruction) of adipocytes.[13] Ghrelin also induces the secretion of gastric acid and pancreatic enzymes, thereby increasing energy absorption.[14] In other words, if one eats fewer calories, increased ghrelin will act to extract more calories out of the smaller portions of food, such that the body absorbs what it needs for maintaining body weight.

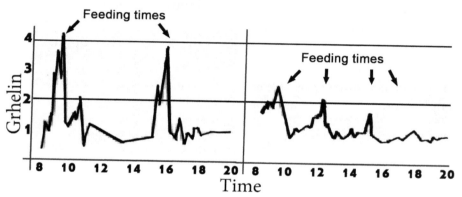

Figure 1-2. Daily ghrelin levels of sheep fed twice per day compared to sheep fed four times per day

Interestingly, total daily ghrelin production doesn't seem to be affected by the number of meals. This is illustrated well in a study in which sheep fed four times a day had ghrelin peaks just before each

---

13   M. S. Kim et al., "The Mitogenic and Antiapoptotic Actions of Ghrelin in 3t3-L1 Adipocytes," *Molecular Endocrinology* (September 2004), http://www.ncbi.nlm.nih.gov/pubmed/15178745.

14   Chih-Yen Chen et al., "Ghrelin Gene Products and the Regulation of Food Intake and Gut Motility," *Pharmacological Reviews* (December 2009), http://pharmrev.aspetjournals.org/content/61/4/430.full#ref-91.

feeding, but the four peaks were not as high as the two peaks of sheep habitually fed only twice a day (figure 1-2).[15] Ghrelin production is increased also via sleep deprivation.[16] And it is suppressed proportionally to the caloric load of the consumed meal.[17]

According to one study, high-protein meals reduce ghrelin more than high-carbohydrate meals.[18] According to another study, carbohydrates appear to be the most effective macronutrient in terms of *immediate* after-meal ghrelin suppression[19] (possibly because of their glucose-elevating and insulin-secreting effect); however, the carbohydrate ingestion provoked a higher ghrelin rise after the meal had been completely absorbed. This second study also therefore concludes that protein is the most satiating macronutrient, as it induces prolonged ghrelin suppression and delay of gastric emptying.

Relative to other carbohydrates, fructose-enriched meals display a poor ghrelin-suppressing capacity, promoting increased caloric intake, weight gain, and obesity under conditions of chronic consumption.

---

15 T. Sugino et al., "A Transient Surge of Ghrelin Secretion before Feeding Is Modified by Different Feeding Regimens in Sheep," *Biochemical and Biophysical Research Communications*, (November 15, 2002), http://www.ncbi.nlm.nih.gov/pubmed/12419323.

16 S. M. Schmid et al., "A Single Night of Sleep Deprivation Increases Ghrelin Levels and Feelings of Hunger in Normal-Weight Healthy Men," *Journal of Sleep Research*, (September 2008), http://www.ncbi.nlm.nih.gov/pubmed/18564298.

17 H. S. Callahan et al., "Postprandial Suppression of Plasma Ghrelin Level Is Proportional to Ingested Caloric Load but Does Not Predict Intermeal Interval in Humans," *Journal of Clinical Endocrinology and Metabolism* (March 2004), http://www.ncbi.nlm.nih.gov/pubmed/15001628.

18 Wendy A. M. Blom et al., "Effect of a High-Protein Breakfast on the Postprandial Ghrelin Response," *American Journal of Clinical Nutrition*, (2006), http://ajcn.nutrition.org/content/83/2/211.full.

19 Chrysi Koliaki et al., "The Effect of Ingested Macronutrients on Postprandial Ghrelin Response: A Critical Review of Existing Literature Data," *International Journal of Peptides* (2010), http://www.hindawi.com/journals/ijpep/2010/710852/.

Leptin

This hormone is primarily produced and released by adipocytes (fat cells), which are like microscopic rubber balloons that can fill up with fat. Leptin powerfully suppresses appetite via the receptors in the hypothalamus. In one study, thirty minutes after injecting leptin into mice, suppression of appetite was induced, lasting more than six hours.[20] *Leptin also increases energy expenditure by burning more fat*, thermogenesis (body temperature), lipid oxidation (fat burning) in brown fat, and lipolysis (breakdown of fat), and it decreases fat synthesis in white and brown fat, leading to a rapid reduction in body weight and adiposity.[21]

When fat levels inside the fat cells are low, they release little to no leptin (figure 1-3). When fat levels inside the cells are normal, normal amounts of leptin are released—the more the cells are filled up and stretched, the more leptin they release. If fat mass remains constant but the number of fat cells increases, each fat cell will contain less fat. Since they are not being stretched, they will release less leptin; therefore, if the total number of fat cells increases with the total fat mass remaining constant, the overall effect is a *decreased* production and release of leptin (figure 1-4).[22]

Leptin is therefore the primary hormone for long-term fat mass homeostasis—as fat mass increases, the release of leptin increases, suppressing appetite and speeding up fat metabolism, bringing the fat mass back down to previous levels. Likewise, as fat mass decreases, the release of leptin decreases, increasing appetite and slowing down fat metabolism, bringing the fat mass back up to previous levels. This explains one of the key difficulties in sustaining weight loss.

---

20 Eric Jéquier and Luc Tappy, "Regulation of Body Weight in Humans," *Physiological Reviews* 79, no. 2 (April 1999), http://physrev.physiology.org/content/79/2/451.
21 U. Sarmiento et al., "Morphologic and Molecular Changes Induced by Recombinant Human Leptin in the White and Brown Adipose Tissues of C57bl/6 Mice," *Laboratory Investigation* (September 1997), http://www.ncbi.nlm.nih.gov/pubmed/9314948.
22 Jéquier and Tappy, "Regulation of Body Weight."

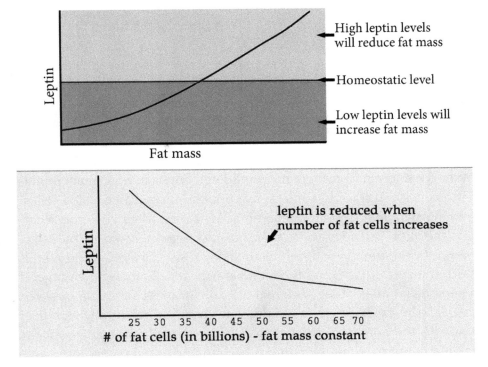

Figure 1-3. (top) Leptin levels in relationship to fat mass

Figure 1-4. (bottom) Leptin levels in relationship to number of fat cells

Interestingly, leptin also strengthens the immune system; one study demonstrates that children with a leptin deficiency have an increased frequency of infections, which is normalized with leptin treatment.[23] This explains how prolonged calorie restriction can lead to illness.

---

23 I. Sadaf Farooqi et al., "Beneficial Effects of Leptin on Obesity: T Cell Hyporesponsiveness, and Neuroendocrine/Metabolic Dysfunction of Human Congenital Leptin Deficiency," *Journal of Clinical Investigation* (October 15, 2002), http://www.ncbi.nlm.nih.gov/pmc/articles/PMC150795/.

HOW CALORIE RESTRICTION ACTUALLY MAKES SOME PEOPLE FATTER

Let's examine how these four hormones interact, taking for example a typical middle-aged person with seventy-five pounds of fat—twenty-five pounds of necessary healthy fat and fifty pounds of excess fat.

Without dieting, his or her total body weight will fluctuate from day to day between two and three pounds and from month to month typically not more than ten to fifteen pounds. Some of that fluctuation is due to changes in water retention and fluctuations in how much food is in the intestinal tract, but at least five pounds of *fat* can be added or lost with normal body-weight fluctuations. However, when you cross a certain threshold outside the *normal fluctuation range of fat mass*—the range of weight variation beyond which the body resists change—leptin levels shift dramatically to bring the fat mass back into homeostatic range. If a person's fat mass changes more drastically from its *homeostatic fat-mass weight*—the exact fat-mass weight that your body naturally stabilizes toward—the hormonal reaction will proportionally change drastically in an attempt to bring the fat mass back to its normal range.

Consider a man who reduces his fat mass beyond his *normal fluctuation range of fat mass*. The automatic reduction in leptin will increase his appetite, conserve energy, and direct metabolism toward fat synthesis. If he pushes himself further, continuing the extreme caloric restriction and further reducing fat mass, the reduced leptin will sacrifice his immune system. This will make him weaker and more susceptible to infection while raising his appetite beyond control and further directing metabolism toward energy conservation and fat synthesis. As soon as he succumbs to hunger and partially increases his caloric intake, his hormonal state will quickly force him to gain back all the fat he lost, while his transformed metabolism will continue with its momentum toward weight gain, even without raising his caloric intake completely back up to what it was before he began his caloric restriction.

All the above effects are solely due to reduced leptin. Now let's examine the additional effects of ghrelin.

Reduced caloric intake will elevate ghrelin levels, increasing hunger and further directing one's metabolism toward fat synthesis, compounding the exact same effects of reduced leptin. Additionally, elevated ghrelin will heighten the secretion of gastric acid and pancreatic enzymes, thereby increasing energy absorption. In other words, one absorbs a greater than normal percentage of calories out of the food digested—sometimes one may eat half the calories that he or she was accustomed to yet not lose any weight!

But here's the catch…*Too much ghrelin over a prolonged time period increases the number of fat cells!* That resets the homeostatic fat-mass set point to a heavier level!

How calorie restriction can actually make people fatter is understood when realizing that the increase in ghrelin increases the number of fat cells, thereby resetting the *homeostatic fat-mass set point* to higher levels. Fat cells "feel" empty unless fat mass is raised proportionally to the higher number of fat cells. The nature of empty fat cells is that they release lesser quantities of leptin, which directs metabolism and hunger to increase fat mass until the fat cells "feel" satisfied.

OTHER FACTORS THAT CAN INCREASE THE NUMBER OF FAT CELLS

An interesting but little-known fact is that *the simultaneous combination of the hormones insulin and cortisol causes an increase in the number of fat cells.* The following descriptions are taken from two studies of fat cells in-vitro (in a test tube), as opposed to in-vivo (live subjects):

1. A thirty- to seventyfold increase in the number of developing fat cells was achieved by the addition of cortisol or related corticosteroids in the presence of insulin. Either of the two hormones alone was ineffective.[24]

---

24 H. Hauner, P. Schmid, and E. F. Pfeiffer, "Glucocorticoids and Insulin Promote the Differentiation of Human Adipocyte Precursor Cells into Fat Cells," *Journal of Clinical Endocrinology and Metabolism*, (April 1987), http://www.ncbi.nlm.nih.gov/pubmed/3546356.

2. Acute amplification of adipose (fat cell) conversion (multiplication) was observed mainly when glucocorticoids (cortisol) and insulin were added simultaneously. Morphological quantification of lipid-containing cells confirmed acceleration of the maturation process.[25]

The reader may be skeptical, since cortisol is released when blood sugar levels are low and insulin is released when blood sugar levels are high. Therefore, the combination of both simultaneously inside human subjects would probably be impossible, right? Wrong! Having simultaneous high levels of both cortisol and insulin is just another paradox of physiology.

If you've been using the mainstream advice *not* to skip breakfast, don't be surprised if you and your patients/clients are getting fatter. Cortisol is at its daily peak half an hour after waking up in the morning. Therefore, if you eat breakfast near that time and if your meal includes carbohydrates that will raise blood sugar levels, not only will your body release insulin to lower the blood sugar levels, but because of the effects of cortisol keeping blood sugar levels high—too high—your body will also be forced to release megadoses of insulin to stabilize your blood sugar. This creates the worst hormonal scenario of simultaneous high levels of both cortisol and insulin, and fat cells will multiply in response. And since empty fat cells don't release the quantities of leptin that we need for fat-mass homeostasis, the *homeostatic fat-mass weight* will be reset to an increased level!

It is correct that people shouldn't "skip" any meal, as doing so raises ghrelin levels as explained above; however, one should never have accustomed oneself to eating an *early* breakfast (ghrelin is released shortly preceding one's *habitual* meal times). According to the Talmud, breakfast should be eaten between three and six hours after waking up. The

---

25 F. Grégoire et al., "Glucocorticoids Induce a Drastic Inhibition of Proliferation and Stimulate Differentiation of Adult Rat Fat Cell Precursors," *Experimental Cell Research* (October 1991), http://www.ncbi.nlm.nih.gov/pubmed/1893938.

important comprehensive physiological benefits of this recommendation are explained in detail in part II: chapters 4 and 7.

What can you do if you are already accustomed to the detrimental habit of eating an early breakfast? You should not suddenly make a drastic change by skipping the meal but rather gradually adapt to delaying breakfast until you are habituated to eating breakfast at least three hours after waking up. For the first couple of weeks, you can try eating a half an hour later, and when that becomes natural and habituated, you can delay breakfast an additional half an hour, and so on.

Additionally, during this transition phase of delaying breakfast, you can reduce inducing insulin secretion and still avoid the damages of elevated ghrelin levels by eating a low-carbohydrate early breakfast consisting of primarily proteins, as protein is most advantageous in the early morning, as explained in detail in chapter 6. Fats and fiber can also subdue ghrelin without spiking insulin. Such a meal will help you avoid high levels of ghrelin by filling your stomach at the habituated time; but by avoiding carbohydrates, you avoid spiking insulin early in the morning when cortisol levels are high. Carbohydrates needed to energize your day can be eaten at a meal three to six hours after waking up.

Alternatively, if for some reason you can't delay breakfast, you can gradually reduce the size of the early breakfast you're accustomed to, replacing those missing calories at a later meal (eaten three to six hours after awakening). Having a prebreakfast snack (less than the size of one mouthful, the equivalent of the volume of an egg)[26] that consists of a small quantity of fruits or vegetables and a small portion of protein one and a half to two hours after waking up is 100 percent acceptable and even recommended by the Talmud.[27] Since cortisol begins to decline from its peak half an hour after you wake up, it won't be so high

26 Rashi's commentary of the Talmud tractate Succah: "A snack as was customary to taste food (the volume of one mouthful) on the way to the study hall" (26A).

27 Talmud tractate Succah: "A snack as was customary to taste food (the volume of one mouthful) on the way to the study hall" (26A). The Tur in chapter 155 of Aruch Chaim writes that it is recommended to have such a snack.

this long after waking up, and such a snack with few carbohydrates and no major protein intake will not invoke much of an insulin response. Therefore, the dangerous conflict of the opposing hormones, cortisol and insulin, won't occur. The advantage of the snack is to avoid the use of body proteins for fuel, as one's glycogen reserves are low after fasting all night, forcing the body to increase the use of other stored energy. Keep in mind that although ingested amino acids (proteins) do not trigger insulin as much as carbohydrates, they do invoke an insulin response.[28] Therefore, the closer in time you are to the cortisol peak (half an hour after waking up), the more careful you need to be to avoid a surge of insulin; thus, if you have a prebreakfast protein snack, it needs to be small and preferably not consumed too early.

Another factor that can raise cortisol levels is stress—emotional and/or physical, not just low blood sugar levels. And if one attempts to comfort oneself when under stress with sweets and other carbohydrates, that will shoot up blood sugar levels and insulin, demonstrating a second scenario that explains the apparent paradox of finding the body loaded with cortisol and insulin simultaneously. This is not at all an uncommon phenomenon. Some people who are desperate to lose weight actually overtrain with too many hours of endurance training or too much of any type of workout, elevating their cortisol levels too high and too long, and then the next meal becomes the bad recipe of cortisol plus insulin yielding more fat cells.

SUMMARY

There are four potent ways to gain fat even when exercising and restricting calories. Although this section (chapter 3) concludes this subject with some solutions to these challenges, I should point out that increasing one's number of fat cells and gaining weight is much easier *and faster* than getting rid of the extra cells and fat.

---

28 N. H. McClenaghan et al., "Mechanisms of Amino Acid-Induced Insulin Secretion from the Glucose-Responsive Brin-Bd11 Pancreatic B-Cell Line," *Journal of Endocrinology* (December 1996), http://www.ncbi.nlm.nih.gov/pubmed/8994380.

To summarize the four processes in which restricting calories can lead to weight gain:

1. **Increased ghrelin**: Restricting calories increases ghrelin, which leads to hunger, fat-synthesizing metabolism, and more efficient extraction of nutrients from digested food.
2. **Decreased leptin**: Restricting calories and reducing body fat leads to a decrease in leptin, leading to hunger, fat-synthesizing metabolism, and a weakened immune system.
3. **Increased number of fat cells from ghrelin**: Too much ghrelin increases the number of fat cells, leading to resetting one's fat-mass homeostasis weight to greater levels, as empty fat cells don't release leptin.
4. **Increased number of fat cells from a combination of insulin and cortisol**: The simultaneous combination of insulin and cortisol also leads to fat cells multiplying, and that happens when one eats an early, high-carbohydrate breakfast or eats carbohydrates under stress.

2

How to Decrease Your Fat Cell Number

FAT CELL APOPTOSIS: OUR SAVIOR

Concerning fat cell number, there is also some good news. You've probably heard that when a person gains weight, the number of fat cells increases, whereas when losing weight, the number of fat cells does not decrease. Well, that's not exactly true. I estimate that the typical reader of this book will have experienced the apoptosis—meaning "death" or "self-destruction"—of approximately 150,000 fat cells in just the fifteen minutes spent on reading the first part of this book.[29]

The bad news is that in those same fifteen minutes, most readers have had the same number or even more new fat cells replace the old ones.

So the key is applying techniques that will maximize fat cell apoptosis while minimizing fat cell reproduction, thereby yielding a steady net decrease in fat cell numbers. The point is that this is possible, and this chapter delves into how to do it.

---

29 The typical lean healthy adult has between twenty-five and thirty billion fat cells. A typical middle-aged, overweight person has about double that, and some extremely obese people can have as many as 250 billion fat cells. The normal lifespan of a fat cell is approximately 8.5 years. Roughly 10 percent of one's fat cells die/self-destruct and are replaced each year. Ten percent of fifty billion fat cells (amount of a typical overweight, middle-aged person) is five billion fat cells. If we divide that by 365 days per year, we get roughly fourteen million; when we divide this number by twenty-four hours, we get roughly six hundred thousand. So in a quarter hour, a person with fifty billion fat cells experiences the apoptosis of roughly one hundred and fifty thousand fat cells.

THE OVERWHELMING POWER
OF GHRELIN AND LEPTIN

For years, fat loss has been perceived as being dependent on willpower and self-discipline. In reality, oftentimes strict discipline and determination can lead people to worsen their health and fitness, when they fight against the nature of their physiology. Our hormones control our long-term fat mass. Success in long-term fat loss only comes with the "consent" of one's hormones. This is best illustrated by examining long-term studies on morbidly obese subjects who underwent a surgical procedure known as sleeve gastrectomy, in which the stomach is reduced to about 25 percent of its original size.

With the stomach so reduced, its capacity to produce ghrelin is also reduced to 25 percent of previous capabilities. However, in actuality, the stomach ends up producing and releasing much less than 25 percent of the amount of ghrelin it was accustomed to presurgery, because stretching the stomach with food consumption stops ghrelin production and release, and such a tiny stomach almost always thinks it's full.

However, shortly after surgery, the stomach begins growing and enlarging, and usually within two years after surgery, it gets big enough to produce enough ghrelin to get back on the old track of weight gain.

A common body weight for people opting for this surgery is around 310 pounds and a BMI of 50. As elaborated above, when losing fat mass, individual fat cells automatically seek to regain homeostatic fat mass by lowering leptin production and release. Therefore, what is so amazing about the success of the typical sleeve gastrectomy subject is that the weight just keeps coming off and off and off for two years, despite the billions of empty fat cells and lack of leptin. That is primarily due to the power of the lack of ghrelin.

A mega-analysis of sixteen studies of 492 subjects[30] shows that the typical 310-pound subject (height 5'7"; BMI 50) will reach a weight as

---

30   Theodoros Diamantis et al., "Review of Long-Term Weight Loss Results after Laparoscopic Sleeve Gastrectomy," *Journal of Surgery for Obesity and Related Diseases* (January–February 2014), Volume 10, Issue 1, Pages 177–183 http://www.soard.org/article/S1550-7289(13)00381-X/fulltext.

low as 175 pounds at the two-year mark after surgery (a loss of 77% of *excess* body weight; BMI 27.4). Then the weight will gradually begin the climb up, such that seven to eight years after surgery he or she is up to 235 pounds (BMI 37).

In review, the typical BMI changes from:
50 before the operation, to
27.4 two years after the operation, to
37 seven years after.

The ten-point increase in BMI roughly equating to regaining sixty pounds is clearly due to the power of leptin. The lack of ghrelin during the first two years after surgery, combined with the long-term reduction in fat mass, will naturally lead the body to reduce the total number of fat cells; however, that process of fat cell reduction is very slow, such that after eight years of reduced ghrelin and body weight, the total number of fat cells could be reduced by 40 to 50 percent, and that is what enables the body to finally stabilize itself at a new homeostatic body weight of 235 pounds compared to the presurgery weight of 310 pounds.

SPEEDING UP APOPTOSIS AND MINIMIZING NEW FAT CELLS

In practical terms, to reach the goal of long-term fat-mass reduction, we need to focus on two goals dreadfully overlooked in the field of dietetics:

1. Speeding up apoptosis of fat cells as much as possible
2. Minimizing the formation of new fat cells as much as possible

In order to speed up apoptosis and inhibit the proliferation of fat cells:

1. Sunbathe
2. Load up on healthy cultured yogurt, cottage cheese, and fish (particularly sardines)
3. Eat plenty of carrots

Alternatively, you can take the following supplements:

1. Vitamin D
2. Calcium
3. Vitamin A

FAT CELL APOPTOSIS VIA VITAMINS A AND D AND CALCIUM

These three nutrients are essential for destroying *old* fat cells (and vitamin A also represses the reproduction of *new* fat cells). Here's the conclusion of one recent study done in June 2014: "High vitamin D and Calcium intakes activate the Calcium (2+)–mediated apoptotic pathway in adipose tissue. The combination of D3 plus Calcium was more effective than D3 or Calcium alone in decreasing adiposity."[31]

Another study comes to essentially the same conclusion, stressing the importance of *high doses* of vitamin D and calcium.[32]

The above two studies are on mice and in vitro. A recent study on four hundred humans confirmed that vitamin D supplementation in deficient humans assists in fat loss.[33] Likewise in another study on humans, calcium supplementation alone (without vitamin D supplementation) demon-

---

31 I. N. Sergeev and Q. Song, "High Vitamin D and Calcium Intakes Reduce Diet-Induced Obesity in Mice By Increasing Adipose Tissue Apoptosis," *Molecular Nutrition and Food Research* (June 2014), http://www.ncbi.nlm.nih.gov/pubmed/24449427.

32 X. Sun and M. B. Zemel, "Role of Uncoupling Protein 2 (UCP 2) Expression and 1Alpha, 25-Dihydroxyvitamin D3 In Modulating Adipocyte Apoptosis," *FASEB Journal* (September 2004), http://www.ncbi.nlm.nih.gov/pubmed/15231722.

33 Vigna et al. "Vitamin D Supplementation Promotes Weight Loss and Waist Circumference Reduction in Overweight/Obese Adults with Hypovitaminosis D," Presented at: European Congress on Obesity. (May 2015); Prague. http://www.clinicaladvisor.com/web-exclusives/vitamin-d-weight-loss-obese-overweight-deficiency/article/413772/

strated a small contribution to fat loss,[34] leaving open the possibility that in combination with vitamin D, the benefits of calcium for humans may be significant. Keep in mind, however, that according to the conclusion of meta-analysis published in 2010,[35] taking calcium supplements alone without coadministered vitamin D is associated with an increased risk of heart attack for women over forty. These findings, however, have been disputed by a more recent study in 2014[36] concluding that calcium supplement intake does not increase the risk of cardiovascular disease in women.

VITAMIN A'S IMPACT ON FAT MASS AND CELL NUMBERS

According to the following study and mega-analysis (on rats, not humans):[37]

"Feeding a high but non-toxic dose of vitamin A (129 mg/kg diet) resulted in a significant reduction in the adiposity index and retroperitoneal white adipose tissue (RPWAT) weight in obese rats while a marginal reduction was observed in lean rats. The feeding of a vitamin A-deficient diet to rats resulted in increased adiposity and body weight gain. Recent studies substantiate the concept that adipocyte deletion by apoptosis is a significant contributor to the regulation of adipose tissue mass and its loss during weight reduction. Retroperitoneal adipose tissue cell density data clearly showed that chronic vitamin

---

34 S. A. Shapses, S. Heshka, and S. B. Heymsfield, "Effect of Calcium Supplementation on Weight and Fat Loss in Women," *Journal of Clinical Endocrinology and Metabolism*, (Feb 2004), http://www.ncbi.nlm.nih.gov/pubmed/14764774.

35 Mark J. Bolland et al., "Effect of Calcium Supplements on Risk of Myocardial Infarction and Cardiovascular Events: Meta-Analysis," *BMJ*, (December 2010), http://www.bmj.com/content/341/bmj.c3691.

36 J. M. Paik et al., "Calcium Supplement Intake and Risk of Cardiovascular Disease in Women," *Osteoporosis International*, (August 2014), http://www.ncbi.nlm.nih.gov/pmc/articles/PMC4102630/.

37 S. M. Jeyakumar et al., "Vitamin A Supplementation Induces Adipose Tissue Loss through Apoptosis in Lean but Not in Obese Rats of the WNIN/OB Strain," *Journal of Molecular Endocrinology* (October 1, 2005), http://jme.endocrinology-journals.org/content/35/2/391.full.

A challenging through diet had no impact on cell size. This formed the basis for our hypothesis that vitamin A-mediated loss of adipose tissue could be through altered (decreased) adipocyte number rather than size."

In addition to carrots, other tasty, healthy, potent sources of vitamin A include sweet potatoes, dark-green leafy vegetables, sweet red peppers, squash, and pink grapefruit. Nonplant sources high in vitamin A include such foods as eggs, dairy, and fish. In addition, adequate intake of dietary protein, fat, and zinc is necessary for the absorption and utilization of vitamin A. (Technically, vitamin A is retinol, and retinol is only found in nonplant sources; plant sources contain carotenoids that the body converts to retinol. Therefore, with plant sources, there is no risk of vitamin A toxicity).

ADDITIONAL CHANNELS VIA WHICH CALCIUM REDUCES FAT MASS

A number of studies[38, 39] have demonstrated that increased dietary calcium reduces fat mass by an additional three mechanisms:

1. Causes fat cells to accelerate lipolysis (fat breakdown) and inhibit lipogenesis (fat buildup)
2. Binds more fatty acids in the colon, thereby inhibiting fat absorption
3. Increases thermogenesis (speeds up metabolism)

Both of these studies claim that dairy-based sources of calcium exert a significantly greater anti-obesity effect than supplemental sources (possibly due to the effects of other bioactive compounds, such as the angiotensin-converting enzyme inhibitor found in milk).

---

38 M. B. Zemel, "Regulation of Adiposity and Obesity Risk by Dietary Calcium: Mechanisms and Implications," *Journal of the American College of Nutrition* (April 2002), http://www.ncbi.nlm.nih.gov/pubmed/11999543.

39 Sarina Schrager, "Dietary Calcium Intake and Obesity," *Journal of the American Board of Family Medicine* (May 2005), http://www.jabfm.org/content/18/3/205.full.

VITAMIN D REDUCES FAT MASS BY IMPROVING INSULIN SENSITIVITY

Vitamin D has also been shown to normalize insulin secretion in patients with impaired insulin secretion, and numerous studies[40, 41] have claimed that it improves insulin sensitivity via at least four avenues:

1. Improved transport of glucose into the muscle
2. Regulation of the nuclear peroxisome-proliferative-activated receptor
3. Stimulation of the expression of insulin receptors[42]
4. Regulation of extracellular calcium, thereby establishing normal calcium inflow through cell membranes and an adequate intracellular cytosolic calcium pool, which is necessary for the insulin-mediated intracellular process in insulin-responsive tissues[43]

For overweight people, improved insulin sensitivity translates into less body fat. This is explained in depth in part II: chapters 4 through 9.

VITAMINS A AND D AND CALCIUM ARE INSUFFICIENT IN THE TYPICAL DIET

In their 2015 report for the US Department of Health, the DGAC (Dietary Guidelines Advisory Committee) characterized these as shortfall nutrients: vitamin A, vitamin D, vitamin E, vitamin C, folate, calcium, magnesium, fiber, and potassium. Of the shortfall nutrients,

---

40 Jessica A. Alvarez and Ambika Ashraf, "Role of Vitamin D in Insulin Secretion and Insulin Sensitivity for Glucose Homeostasis," *International Journal of Endocrinology* (2010), http://www.ncbi.nlm.nih.gov/pmc/articles/PMC2778451/.

41 Afsaneh Talaei, Mahnaz Mohamadi, and Zahra Adgi, "The Effect of Vitamin D on Insulin Resistance in Patients with Type 2 Diabetes," *Diabetology and Metabolic Syndrome* (2013), http://www.dmsjournal.com/content/5/1/8.

42 Sedigheh Soheilykhah, "The Role of Adipocyte Mediators, Inflammatory Markers and Vitamin D in Gestational Diabetes," *Intech* (November 2011), http://cdn.intechopen.com/pdfs-wm/23178.pdf.

43 Ibid.

calcium, vitamin D, fiber, and potassium also are classified as nutrients of public health concern because their underconsumption has been linked in scientific literature to adverse health outcomes. Furthermore, the DGAC writes that the typical intake is too high for refined grains, added sugars, sodium, and saturated fat.

LEPTIN RESISTANCE

So far I explained how the hormone leptin reduces body fat via directing metabolism away from fat synthesis toward fat burning and appetite suppression. And I explained how to increase leptin by decreasing the number of fat cells. But if the body is *resistant* to leptin, leptin won't be effective in its job of reducing fat.

The more leptin our fat cells release, the slimmer we get. Therefore, one would assume that slim people have loads of leptin, and that's what keeps them slim, while fat people lack it, and their problem is leptin deficiency. However, leptin deficiency is a very rare phenomenon. The vast majority of obese people have much more leptin than thin people, as greater fat mass produces more leptin; however, their bodies are "resistant" to the slimming effects of leptin.[44]

Leptin resistance is another challenge to take into consideration when designing a plan to combat obesity. It should also be observed that leptin resistance gets worse with age,[45] making it more difficult to reduce body fat as we get older. There are theories as to what may contribute to leptin resistance, but so far there is no known "golden" solution to this problem.

---

44 Eric Jéquier and Luc Tappy, "Regulation of Body Weight in Humans," *Physiological Reviews*, (April 1999), http://physrev.physiology.org/content/79/2/451.
45 Z. W. Wang et al., "The Role of Leptin Resistance in the Lipid Abnormalities of Aging," *FASEB Journal*, (January 2001), http://www.ncbi.nlm.nih.gov/pubmed/11149898.

3

Customizing Your Fat-Mass Reduction Plan

PLANNING PERSONAL PACING FOR FAT LOSS TO ENSURE LONG-TERM SUCCESS

This book supplies the best-known methods for fat reduction, both short term and long term, but to attain the greatest success, it is important to be realistic about one's fat-loss goals. If one loses weight too fast, the lack of leptin will slow one's metabolism and weaken his or her immune system, inevitably making long-term fat loss slower and more difficult. This is a very important point that cannot be stressed enough. Unfortunately, what is most popular are the diets that promise (and deliver) the fastest and biggest short-term results. But when not pacing weight loss properly according to one's individual abilities, the results are usually harmful in the long run.

A combination of numerous factors determines an individual's fastest long-term weight-loss pace. This section attempts to provide the information that enables you to figure out how to pace yourself properly. In practical terms, you will need to experiment with the most effective short-term weight loss methods and then set your pace for weight loss according to your individual situation, based on the following guide.

The speed of long-term weight loss varies between individuals. You might ask, Why do I need to know what factors affect this speed? The answer is that you should know this in order to gauge a speed appropriate for you.

25

To illustrate, let's compare two middle-aged persons of the same gender and equal body compositions (fat mass relative to muscle mass, height, and weight). For purposes of illustration, let's call our test subjects Moe and Larry. Both were at their ideal weight at age twenty. The difference between them is that Moe maintained his ideal weight right up until half a year ago, when all of a sudden, a tragedy befell him, and the emotional stress led him to put on fifty pounds of fat in the last six months. Larry, on the other hand, began gaining two to three pounds per year since age twenty. It should be obvious that Moe will much more easily knock off those extra fifty pounds and could possibly do so in the same time that he gained it, while Larry will hit a plateau as soon as he knocks off ten pounds, and if he pushes himself to try and lose more, he will get sick and immediately put back all the weight he lost and more.

What is the physiological reason behind their differences? Each year that Larry added on another two to three pounds, his body adapted by increasing the number of fat cells; that increased his *homeostatic fat-mass weight* each year in proportion to the weight he gained. In contrast, Moe's *homeostatic fat-mass weight*—the exact fat-mass weight that your body naturally stabilizes toward—could not possibly change from twenty-five pounds to seventy-five pounds in just six months' time.

If both Moe and Larry had twenty-five billion fat cells at age twenty, Moe still has close to that amount; perhaps in the last six months they rose 5 to 10 percent to between twenty-six and twenty-seven billion, while Larry probably added on 5 to 10 percent of fat cells per year over a period of twenty years and thus accumulated over fifty billion fat cells by now.

Moe, with merely twenty-six to twenty-seven billion fat cells, is now loaded with leptin, because all of his fat cells are extremely stretched out, holding almost triple the fat mass that they are accustomed to in their homeostatic state, causing the fat cells to release megadoses of leptin. That means that without any dieting effort at all, just by merely stopping the emotionally induced compulsive overeating, Moe will automatically drop back down almost completely to his previous weight, just through the powerful effects of high levels of leptin. Being overweight six months has just slightly expanded his number of fat cells and just slightly raised his *homeostatic fat-mass weight* from twenty-five pounds to perhaps *twenty-seven pounds*.

In contrast, Larry, with over fifty billion fat cells, has just enough leptin to maintain the status quo. His *homeostatic fat-mass weight* is now *seventy-five pounds*, as he has gradually reached this weight over a twenty-year period.

HOW SHOULD THE FAT-LOSS PLAN BE INDIVIDUALIZED FOR EACH PERSON?

This question seems to be ignored in all the diets I have studied: the Dukan Diet, the American Heart Association's No-Fad Diet, Atkins, South Beach, Dr. Barry Sear's Zone, Paleo, Dr. Fuhrman's Eat to Live, Mark Macdonald's Body Confidence, and more.

Yet this personalized analysis needs to be the very foundation in planning for an individual's fat-loss program. This is not a secret teaching of Maimonides or the Talmud. It is the most basic application of physiology in regard to weight-loss diets. The following is a formula for planning a pace for fat loss that is appropriate for each *individual*—how to set the ideal pace leading to the fastest, greatest, and most permanent success:

1. Increase intake of calcium and vitamins D and A. Currently, there is insufficient information concerning fat cell apoptosis to know the fastest-possible rate of reducing one's fat cell number. But the method of doing it naturally is clear: high doses of calcium and vitamins D and A, combined with sustained fat loss.
2. Follow the healthiest and fastest fat-loss methods, as explained in chapter 16.
3. Each person will need to experiment with short-term weight loss until he or she discovers *the point at which the body resists fat loss*. For some individuals, this could be after a week and a loss of three pounds of water and three pounds of fat; for others, it could be after a month and a loss of four pounds of water and

twenty pounds of fat or even more. In our example, Larry can expect to lose between five and ten pounds of fat before encountering stiff hormonal resistance.

4. Once you reach your personal fat-loss resistance point, you need to change over from a weight-loss diet to a weight-maintenance diet, continuing to take plenty of calcium and vitamins D and A. You should expect a slow drift upward in your weight since you are now a few pounds below your homeostatic fat-mass weight. Since there are normal weight fluctuations from hour to hour and day to day, you need to carefully keep track of your waistline with a body tape measure every morning to ensure that you don't drift back up to your previous fat-mass homeostatic weight. Therefore, on most days you should eat healthy foods *freely* according to your appetite, according to the long-term maintenance plan of Maimonides and the Talmud (as explained in part II: chapters 4 through 9). Only one or two days a week, switch to a healthy fat-loss diet (as explained in chapter 16) in order to counter the natural upward drift toward your homeostatic fat-mass weight.

     Eventually your number of fat cells will drop (due to lowered fat mass plus increased vitamins A and D and calcium), and you will have successfully reset your homeostatic fat-mass weight to your current lower weight. This stabilization period could last from two to twelve weeks, depending on the individual and his or her particular set of circumstances.

5. Then, you switch back to the fat-loss diet plan until you reach the next plateau. And, unlike the advice of many popular diets on the market, don't try to push yourself beyond your *normal fluctuation range of fat mass* (to be explained shortly). If you do, your body will fight back harder than you, and you will end up resetting your homeostatic fat-mass weight to a higher level as explained in the beginning of part I. Rather, be patient and switch over to the fat-mass maintenance diet, eating healthy

foods freely according to your appetite, tracking your new smaller waistline, and ensuring that you don't drift back up to your previous homeostatic fat-mass weight by switching to the healthy fat-loss diet one or two days a week.

Eventually your fat cell numbers will drop further, and you will have once again successfully reset your homeostatic fat-mass weight to your current lower weight. Once your weight is stabilized so that you don't need to switch to the fat-loss diet to maintain your new lower weight, then you can strive again for weight loss until reaching yet a lower new plateau.

NORMAL FLUCTUATION RANGE OF FAT MASS

As illustrated above, the *fat-mass homeostasis weight*—the fat-mass weight that your body naturally stabilizes toward—largely depends on how long it took for you to gain that fat and how many fat cells you have. But you also need to consider your *normal fluctuation range of fat mass*—the range of weight variation that beyond which the body resists change. Now to explain how this range is proportional to your total fat mass:

As an example, we'll continue with our test subject Larry, having seventy-five pounds of fat mass. One would expect his *normal fluctuation range of fat mass* to be around 10 percent of his total fat mass—7.5 pounds.

Let's compare him to our third test subject, Curly. Curly is also middle aged and also spent twenty years gradually gaining fat; however, Curly has 150 pounds of fat, compared to Larry, who has seventy-five. With 150 pounds of fat, all else being equal, Curly would expect his *normal fluctuation range of fat mass* to be around a loss of 10 percent of that, or 15 pounds, compared to Larry's of 7.5 pounds. Reducing fat mass by more than the *normal fluctuation range of fat mass* will invoke stiff hormonal resistance, doing more harm than good.

Of course, other factors also determine one's *homeostasis fat-mass weight* and *normal fluctuation range of fat mass*, such as genetics, gender, age, physical and emotional stresses, and one's physical health condition.

With patience, this plan will lead to sustained weight loss, because you'll be focusing on lowering your number of fat cells and your *homeostatic fat-mass weight*, as opposed to ignoring these ultimate determining factors by focusing merely on weight loss, which often raises fat cell number and one's *homeostatic fat-mass weight*.

TO LOSE WEIGHT OR NOT TO LOSE WEIGHT: THAT IS NOT THE QUESTION

I sometimes ask overweight individuals how they would prefer to see themselves a year from now: "Assuming that your waist size will be exactly the same as it is today, would you prefer to see yourself ten pounds heavier or ten pounds lighter?"

The inevitable response is "ten pounds lighter." But that is wrong!

If your waist size stays the same, but you've lost ten pounds, you haven't lost fat but rather muscle. And if you gained ten pounds and your waist size stays the same, you haven't gained fat but rather muscle.

Many people find this confusing, questioning, "Wouldn't weight loss automatically entail a trimmer waistline?"

A friend of mine who manages the local health food store is in need of a liver transplant. Recently his situation got so bad that he stopped coming to work. I bumped into him in the post office, and his complexion was gray-green. He had lost a lot of weight since the last time I had seen him. His arms and legs were just thin bones. He said he was so weak that he could hardly pull himself out of bed to manage the details required to get his insurance company to cover the transplant. But his stomach was bloated—a much bigger waistline than the last time I saw him. So the short answer: "No. Weight loss does not automatically entail a trimmer waistline."

Generally, when people lose weight, it entails a loss of fat (primarily from the waistline), but also a loss of water, glycogen reserves, and muscle. Temporarily reducing water and glycogen reserves is usually not a problem; in fact, as I explain in chapter 16, lower glycogen reserves help speed up fat loss. But muscle loss is bad. Over the long term, water and glycogen fluctuations are negligible. The more enduring body changes are in fat and muscle mass. Muscle mass change is most noticeable in leg and arm width as well as chest size, whereas stronger stomach muscles do not equate to a larger waistline. Changes in fat mass do occur in other parts of the body, but primarily influence waistline size (and hip size for women).

The most effective way to increase muscle mass is to lift heavy weights with appropriate diet and rest. And the quickest way to lose muscle mass is to fast or go on an extremely low-calorie diet.

When people fast or nearly fast, most of their weight loss comes from consumed muscle mass, and only a smaller portion is fat loss. Surely their waistline will be a little smaller. But if they gain back some weight when they increase their caloric intake, the regained weight can be nearly all fat. In such a case, they could *regain* all the *fat* they lost, while remaining ten pounds lighter due to the *muscle* they lost—not good.

If a man put on ten pounds of muscle over a year of heavy weight lifting, it's possible he gained some fat during that type of training, raising his weight by a few pounds of fat in addition to the ten pounds of muscle. But if he then reverts to an aerobic training program and a well-designed fat-loss diet, he can get rid of those gained pounds of fat and more. If the net result is ten pounds heavier due to added muscle, with no change in fat mass, his waistline will be just what it was before he put on the ten pounds of muscle.

The point is to focus on fat loss as opposed to weight loss.

THE METABOLIC ADVANTAGE OF MUSCLE

Muscle is a very valuable asset. Men are usually more interested in being muscular than women; many women are afraid of "bulking up" with muscle mass. Often women don't realize that the strength training that leads female Olympic runners, skaters, swimmers, and gymnasts to become much stronger and more muscular than the average woman doesn't necessarily cause them to become bulky. In truth, stronger and more muscular isn't always bulkier—especially for women as compared to men, as women typically have less testosterone and more difficulty in gaining substantial muscle mass.

Muscle is denser than fat, occupying roughly 80 percent of the volume (space) of the same amount of fat. This means that in comparing two women of the same weight, the more muscular one will be thinner. Even when comparing two women of equal volume (whom would both displace the same amount of water out of a completely filled tank of water), even though the more muscular woman will weigh more, she will be more shapely and toned.

But beyond aesthetics, muscle has many health benefits, including metabolic benefits. The body burns calories just to sustain muscle mass—even when sleeping. In contrast, maintaining fat mass requires virtually no energy. In fact, during sleep, the calories recruited for muscle sustenance come primarily from fat reserves.

Too many people smile at their imagined success when gazing at the scales and think that the weight they have lost is an achievement. Too often, following poor nutritional advice, a large portion of the weight loss comes from muscle, making their body weak and sagging. Ninety percent of these people end up regaining the lost weight partly due to a slowed-down metabolism, but they end up fatter and weaker than prior due to misguided efforts.

I've even occasionally seen before-and-after pictures where the subject really believes that he or she looks better after losing muscle mass due to the massive body-volume reduction, not realizing that those pictures actually display the proportions of a person obviously dramatically weaker—a drooping bag of bones.

So put the focus on your waist measurement more than the weight scale. Women can also keep tabs on their hip measurement to monitor fat-loss progress. And focus on overall health and fitness, while striving for long term *fat* loss (as opposed to *weight* loss), via patiently lowering your homeostatic fat-mass weight.

Part II

The Metabolic Syndrome

Obesity, Prediabetes, and Heart Disease: Developing Lifelong Habits for Better Health and Insulin Sensitivity

4

The Metabolic Syndrome: Its Causes and Remedies

The metabolic syndrome—a combination of obesity and high cholesterol, blood pressure, and blood sugar—increases the risk of heart disease, cancer, and diabetes, some of the leading causes of death. The prevalence of this syndrome is estimated to be between 20 and 25 percent of adult Americans![46]

This chapter delves deeply into how our bodies work in order to understand the causes and remedies of the metabolic syndrome. This chapter includes the following subjects:

- What is the Metabolic Syndrome?
- Insulin Resistance and Hyperinsulinemia: the Root of the Metabolic Syndrome
- Atherosclerosis and the Metabolic Syndrome
- Root of Insulin Resistance
- Overconsumption of Carbohydrates Is Converted to Body Fat
- The Liver: Storing Fat or Burning Fat
- How Hyperinsulinemia Perpetuates Itself
- Hyperinsulinemia Equals More Fat Cells Equals Increased Fat Mass
- The Maimonides Cure for Hyperinsulinemia

---

46 American Heart Association, http://www.heart.org/idc/groups/heart-public/@wcm/@hcm/documents/downloadable/ucm_300322.pdf.

WHAT IS THE METABOLIC SYNDROME?

A person who has at least three of the following conditions is defined as having the metabolic syndrome:[47]

1. *A large waistline*: Also called abdominal obesity or "having an apple shape." Excess fat in the stomach area (a greater than thirty-five-inch waist for women and forty-inch waist for men) presents a greater risk factor for heart disease than excess fat in other parts of the body, such as on the hips.
2. *A high triglyceride level (or taking medicine to treat high triglycerides)*: Triglycerides are a type of fat found in the blood.
3. *A low HDL cholesterol level* (or taking medicine to treat low HDL cholesterol)*: HDL is sometimes called "good" cholesterol because it helps remove cholesterol from one's arteries. A low HDL cholesterol level raises the risk for heart disease.
4. *High blood pressure* (or taking medicine to treat high blood pressure)*.
5. *High fasting blood sugar* (or taking medicine to treat high blood sugar)*: Mildly high blood sugar may be an early sign of diabetes.

* See the end of the last chapter for parameters.

The risk for heart disease, diabetes, and stroke increases with the number of metabolic risk factors one has. In general, *a person who has the metabolic syndrome is twice as likely to develop heart disease and five times as likely to develop diabetes as someone who doesn't have the metabolic syndrome.*[48]

Other risk factors also increase the risk for heart disease, but they aren't part of the metabolic syndrome; for example, high LDL (bad) cholesterol level and smoking.

---

47 National Heart Lung and Blood Institute of the US Department of Health and Human Services, National Institutes of Health, http://www.nhlbi.nih.gov/health/health-topics/topics/ms/.
48 Ibid.

Having even one risk factor raises the risk for heart disease. The risk of having metabolic syndrome is closely linked to obesity, a lack of physical activity, and insulin resistance.

INSULIN RESISTANCE AND HYPERINSULINEMIA: THE ROOT OF THE METABOLIC SYNDROME

Hyperinsulinemia—having too much insulin—and insulin resistance are considered the root causes of the metabolic syndrome. One of the main functions of insulin is to transfer excess sugar from the blood into the liver and muscle cells. When cells are said to be resistant to insulin, it means that they resist the transfer of sugar. Thus the sugar remains in the blood, and glucose levels remain higher than they should be. This causes the body to release more and more insulin in an attempt to lower blood sugar to safe levels. This excess of insulin secretion is called *hyperinsulinemia*. For people with glucose levels that are too high because of insulin resistance but not as high as type 2 diabetes, the term *prediabetes* is used.

According to the American Heart Association, insulin-resistance/ hyperinsulinemia alone (even without obesity) is implicated in the development of hypertension and atherosclerotic cardiovascular disease.[49] It is assumed that this happens via abnormalities in insulin signaling and associated cardiovascular and metabolic derangements. In other words, insulin resistance and hypertension are interrelated processes.

Additionally, as previously discussed, insulin-resistance/hyperinsulinemia causes higher levels of cholesterol, because insulin increases the enzyme HMG-CoA reductase,[50] which is the enzyme responsible for

---

49 Julia Steinberger and Stephen R. Daniels, "Obesity, Insulin Resistance, Diabetes, and Cardiovascular Risk in Children," *Circulation Journal*, American Heart Association, (2003). http://circ.ahajournals.org/content/107/10/1448.long

50 G. C. Ness and C. M. Chambers, "Feedback and Hormonal Regulation of Hepatic 3-Hydroxy-3-Methylglutaryl Coenzyme A Reductase: The Concept of Cholesterol Buffering Capacity," *Proceedings of the Society for Experimental Biology and Medicine* 224, no. 1 (May 2000): 8–19, http://www.ncbi.nlm.nih.gov/pubmed/10782041.

causing the liver to produce cholesterol.[51] (Statins are a drug that lowers LDL cholesterol levels by inhibiting this enzyme.) In fact, most people produce four times more cholesterol in their liver than they ingest with their food. That means that even if one eats a low-cholesterol diet, he or she will still have high cholesterol if his or her blood sugar levels are high.

Hyperinsulinemia is also directly responsible for obesity, as explained shortly. And obesity increases the risk of high blood pressure. *So as we see, the root cause of the metabolic syndrome is hyperinsulinemia: too much insulin.* And the root cause of hyperinsulinemia is insulin resistance, where the body responds slowly and only to large amounts of insulin before lowering blood sugar.

ATHEROSCLEROSIS AND THE METABOLIC SYNDROME

Atherosclerosis results from high LDL cholesterol, a symptom that can be related to the metabolic syndrome. Atherosclerosis—clogging of the arteries—is the usual cause of heart attacks, strokes, and peripheral vascular disease (clogging of peripheral arteries). Atherosclerotic cardiovascular disease is the number one killer in the adult population of Western societies.[52]

Atherosclerosis begins with damage to the endothelium caused by high blood pressure, smoking, or high cholesterol and leads to plaque formation. The endothelium is the thin layer of cells that line the arteries—the blood vessels that carry blood from the heart throughout the body. The endothelium work to keep the inside of the arteries toned and smooth and to keep the blood flowing.

When "bad" cholesterol, or LDL, crosses a damaged endothelium, cholesterol enters the wall of the artery. This causes white blood cells to stream in to digest the LDL. Over years, the accumulation of cholesterol and white blood cells becomes plaque in the wall of the artery.

---

51 W. Wang and T. J. Tong, "The Key Enzyme of Cholesterol Synthesis Pathway: HMG-COA Reductase and Disease," *Sheng Li Ke Xue Jin Zhan* 30, no. 1 (January 1999): 5–9.

52 Julia Steinberger and Stephen R. Daniels, "Obesity, Insulin Resistance, Diabetes."

Plaque is a mixture of cholesterol, cells, and debris that creates a bump on the artery wall. As atherosclerosis progresses, that bump gets bigger. When it gets big enough, it can create a blockage. That process goes on throughout the entire body. The plaques of atherosclerosis cause the three main kinds of cardiovascular disease: heart attacks, strokes, and poor leg circulation, causing pain when walking, which can become a cause for amputation.

ROOT OF INSULIN RESISTANCE
To understand what causes insulin resistance and how to make the body more sensitive to insulin, it is necessary to have a basic understanding of the hormones involved, their effects on the liver, and the liver's contribution to blood sugar levels.

Since the brain doesn't store energy, to keep itself alive and functioning it depends primarily upon sugar in the blood. Between meals, when the sugar in the blood gets used up, the hormones—epinephrine, norepinephrine and cortisol (all three produced by the adrenal glands) and glucagon (produced in the pancreas)—affect the liver and cause it to release sugar into the blood. The average adult male's liver can store approximately 110 grams of glycogen, equivalent to 440 calories. These hormones also direct fat cells to release fat for energy into the bloodstream and direct the liver to convert fat and protein into glucose.

The average adult male's capacity to store carbohydrates is limited to about 450 grams—approximately 110 grams in the liver and 340 grams within the muscle mass.[53] What is stored in the muscle cannot

---

53 In the liver cells (hepatocytes), glycogen can compose up to 8 percent of the fresh weight (100–120 grams in an adult) soon after a meal. Only the glycogen stored in the liver can be made accessible to other organs. In the muscles, glycogen is found in a low concentration (1–2 percent of the muscle mass). The amount of glycogen stored in the body—especially within the muscles, liver, and red blood cells—depends primarily on physical training, basal metabolic rate, and eating habits such as intermittent fasting. Small amounts of glycogen are found in the kidneys, and even smaller amounts in certain glial cells in the brain and white blood cells. The uterus also stores glycogen during pregnancy to nourish the embryo.

transfer to the blood and the rest of the body but rather can only be used by the muscles.

OVERCONSUMPTION OF CARBOHYDRATES IS CONVERTED TO BODY FAT

If one eats carbohydrates when his or her body's storage capacity for carbohydrates is already full, all the carbohydrates that are not needed for immediate use will be converted to fat. The opposite end of the spectrum is when glycogen reserves are extremely low (glycogen is glucose altered chemically for storage in the liver and muscles). A person who runs a marathon and completely depletes his or her stores of glycogen will usually need about twenty-four hours for the body to turn enough carbohydrates into glycogen to fully replenish the stores. Normally, when you begin eating a meal, the stores are not completely depleted, and as such, the body can only accept a maximum of two hundred to three hundred grams of carbohydrates. *If one consumes more carbohydrates, they are converted to and stored as fat.*

However, sedentary people who snack between meals typically have their glycogen stores nearly full before starting their meals, in which case the consumption of a mere two hundred calories (fifty grams) of carbohydrates can exceed storage capacity, forcing the body to convert the excess carbohydrates to body fat.

Converting sugar to fat for storage in fat cells—or the reverse, converting fat to sugar to supply the body with energy—takes place in the liver.

THE LIVER: STORING FAT OR BURNING FAT

Question: What determines if your liver is going to store fat or burn it?

The answer depends on which hormones are exerting more influence on the liver: either the *fat-burning* hormones (adrenalin, cortisol, glucagon, and/or growth hormone) or the *fat-storing* hormone insulin. Overweight people need to minimize their amount of insulin, in order to maximize the burning of fat.

HOW HYPERINSULINEMIA PERPETUATES ITSELF

So far I have explained how hyperinsulinemia is the root cause of the metabolic syndrome. Shortly I will explain how the problem of hyper-insulinemia perpetuates itself, but three obvious ways of avoiding it are to

1. eat only a moderate quantity of carbohydrates,
2. choose carbohydrates with a low glycemic index (carbohydrates that are absorbed slowly), and
3. digest the carbohydrates together with fats and fiber to slow the absorption of carbohydrates.[54, 55, 56]

When the blood sugar level rises beyond a certain point after a person eats a meal with carbohydrates, insulin is secreted. These three suggestions will minimize blood sugar spikes and hence minimize the insulin response.

Additionally, if liver or muscle storage space is available for excess sugar in the blood, and there is no insulin resistance, then with a minimal secretion of insulin, the sugar level will be quickly balanced, and the storage facilities in the liver and muscle will be replenished. If excess insulin is avoided, cortisol and glucagon won't be blocked from converting fats to sugars to maintain the needed energy supply as the body burns fuel to sustain itself during the hours after the meal.

But if large quantities of carbohydrates are eaten (especially if they are high-glycemic-index carbohydrates), sugar levels spike, triggering the secretion of much insulin. If storage facilities are full, there will be insulin resistance, meaning that despite the increasing insulin secretion, sugar levels will remain high because there is no place to which to

---

54 D. J. Jenkins et al., "Dietary Fibres, Fibre Analogues, and Glucose Tolerance: Importance of Viscosity," *British Medical Journal*, (1978), http://www.bmj.com/content/1/6124/1392.

55 Institute of Medicine, *Dietary Reference Intakes* (National Academies Press, 2005), 380–82.

56 Sareen S. Gropper, Jack L. Smith, and James L. Groff, *Advanced Nutrition and Human Metabolism*, 5th edition, Cengage Learning 2008), 114.

transfer the sugar outside of the blood, and the high blood sugar levels force the body to continue to secrete more and more insulin.

The excessive insulin then blocks the usage of fats as an energy source for hours to come.[57] Eventually the body manages to lower the excess sugar in the blood by using the blood sugar to fuel the body's energy needs. Blood sugar levels are also reduced by insulin's effect on the liver, directing it to convert sugar into fat. Eventually blood sugar levels drop so low that the body releases hormones to raise its blood sugar; however, these hormones can't be effective because of the excessive insulin still in the system that has the opposite effect. Then, blood sugar levels drop down too low, but because the overload of insulin has not dissipated, the body can't access stored sugars in the liver or stored energy in the fat cells. And with the brain in danger, the body sends out panic signals of hunger for more carbohydrates.

Of course, with the insulin having blocked the release of sugar in the liver, the liver's storage capacity remains full. Therefore, when blood sugar levels spike up again after quenching the ferocious appetite, the sugar can't be stored as glycogen in the liver but rather has to undergo the slow process of being converted to fat in the liver and sent to fat cells for storage. So the cycle of insulin resistance and high levels of insulin secretion continues until the sugar levels are slowly lowered, blocking any usage of fats or even using stored sugar. The blood sugar levels resemble a roller coaster ride, going up and down in extremes, with a nonstop, out-of-control appetite.

HYPERINSULINEMIA YIELDS MORE FAT CELLS WHICH YIELDS INCREASED FAT MASS

Another disastrous outcome of hyperinsulinemia is gaining more fat cells. We just discussed how a small meal can spike insulin secretion when all the storage space for sugar is already full. We also looked at how the high amounts of insulin eventually lead to low blood sugar levels.

---

57 M. E. Valera Mora et al., "Insulin Clearance in Obesity," *Journal of the American College of Nutrition*, (December 2003), http://www.ncbi.nlm.nih.gov/pubmed/14684753.

It's important to understand that once released, insulin doesn't disappear instantaneously once sugar levels drop but rather goes through a process of degradation that takes about an hour after eating a meal in healthy individuals.[58] However, in people with hyperinsulinemia, the process of insulin clearance is impaired, delaying the process further.[59] The excessive insulin that stays in the blood too long frequently leads to blood sugar levels dropping too low. To counter the low blood sugar, the body increases cortisol (among other hormones), which ordinarily gets the sugar levels back up; however, when the blood is overloaded with insulin, cortisol is ineffective, forcing the body to release more and more cortisol.

The blood is then a dangerous soup, overloaded with excessive insulin and cortisol, and it is precisely this paradoxical combination (insulin is released when sugar levels are high, while cortisol is released when sugar levels are low) that signals fat cells to speed up the process of adding more fat cells.[60, 61] Chapter 1 explains in detail how the increase in number of fat cells leads to the reduction of the hormone leptin, which leads to increased fat mass. This chapter shows how hyperinsulinemia compounds these problems.

THE MAIMONIDES CURE FOR HYPERINSULINEMIA

The way out of that cycle is to burn off high levels of blood sugar with physical activity and then to maintain balanced blood sugar levels with *small quantities* of *low-glycemic-index carbohydrates*. Eventually insulin levels will come down, enabling cortisol and glucagon to be effective

---

58 William C. Duckworth, Robert G. Bennett, and Frederick G. Hamel, "Insulin Degradation: Progress and Potential," *Endocrine Reviews* (July 1, 2013), http://press.endocrine.org/doi/full/10.1210/edrv.19.5.0349.

59 Mora et al., "Insulin Clearance in Obesity," *Journal of the American College of Nutrition*, (December 2003), http://www.ncbi.nlm.nih.gov/pubmed/14684753.."

60 H. Hauner, P. Schmid, and E. R. Pfeiffer, "Glucocorticoids and Insulin Promote The Differentiation Of Human Adipocyte Precursor Cells Into Fat Cells," *Journal of Clinical Endocrinology and Metabolism* (April 1987), http://www.ncbi.nlm.nih.gov/pubmed/3546356.

61 F. Grégoire et al., "Glucocorticoids Induce a Drastic Inhibition of proliferation and stimulate differentiation of adult rat fat cell precursors," *Experimental Cell Research* (October 1991), http://www.ncbi.nlm.nih.gov/pubmed/1893938.

in their job of preventing low blood sugar by constantly feeding the blood with a slow and steady supply of energy from stored sugars and fats.

The following are the four primary components of the long-term solution to hyperinsulinemia. They are explained in the following chapters in detail.

1. **Early dinner**: It is crucial to refrain from eating three to four hours before bedtime.[62] Drinking water is fine.

2. **Exercise**: It is especially important to exercise before breakfast.[63]

3. **Late breakfast**: Ideally you should eat your first full meal three to six hours after waking up (a small pre-breakfast snack is recommended).[64] By beginning your daily fast three to four hours before bedtime and continuing it until three to six hours after you wake up, you attain a daily intermittent fast of at least thirteen hours. This break enables your body, assisted by nighttime hormones, to burn fats in the most natural way and ensures that the body will be receptive to insulin at breakfast time, breaking the cycle of hyperinsulinemia. Intermittent fasting also has cleansing and healing benefits that are explained in detail in chapter 9.

4. **Measured glycemic load**: Whereas the US Department of Health recommends a high carbohydrate consumption of 45 to 65 percent of total calories, and Dr. Atkins recommends an extremely low-carbohydrate diet of less than 10 percent, many doctors today recommend a moderately low-carbohydrate diet (such as Dr. Barry Sears, author of *The Zone Diet*, and Dr. Loren Cordain, author of *The Paleo Diet* (pg. 24), who recommend that carbohydrates should be limited to 40 percent of total caloric intake). To avoid hyperinsulinemia, it is necessary to limit

---

62 Maimonides, Mishna Torah, sefer HaMada, hilchat Dayot, chapter 4, paragraph 5.

63 Ibid., chapter 4, paragraph 2.

64 Talmud, Tractate Pesachim 12b, Tractate Shabbas 10a, and Shulchan Aruch, Aruch Chaim chapter 157. The Mishna Brura writes in the name of the Magen Avroham that the hours mentioned in the Talmud are calculated from the time of waking up.

carbohydrate intake. Dr. Atkins's low recommendation is too difficult for most people to maintain on a permanent basis, but above 40 percent would not be good for diabetics, prediabetics, or for obese individuals with insulin resistance problems.

In general, is preferable to consume carbohydrates with low glycemic indexes and to avoid blood sugar spikes by eating the carbohydrates together with fiber and fats.[65, 66, 67] Your carbohydrate intake should be divided fairly evenly throughout the day, with the biggest portion being consumed in a late breakfast, to provide you with sufficient energy to manage your daily tasks.

It is important that you do not change your dietary habits drastically overnight; if you desire to change them, make gradual changes. For example, if you are accustomed to eating right up until your bedtime, adjust your lifestyle the first week by finishing eating half an hour before bedtime. Then, the second week, stop eating an hour before bed. If you are not accustomed to exercising, then don't go out on the first day and try to run for an hour straight. Rather, walk briskly for fifteen minutes each morning, eventually adding time and speed. If you are accustomed to eating breakfast within a half hour after waking up, don't push off breakfast three hours your first day but rather push it off thirty minutes the first week, and extend the time when you feel comfortable with the changes. Making drastic, sudden changes in your dietary lifestyle is a sure recipe for instability and is almost always harmful to one's health—sometimes extremely harmful. One of the reasons is that the body releases ghrelin at the time it habitually expects a meal, and skipping the meal or delaying it for several hours will prevent the ghrelin levels from subsiding, which leads to hunger, slowed metabolism, and obesity, as explained in detail in chapter 1.

---

65 Jenkins et al., "Dietary Fibres, Fibre Analogues, and Glucose Tolerance: Importance of Viscosity," *British Medical Journal*, (1978), http://www.bmj.com/content/1/6124/1392.

66 Institute of Medicine, *Dietary Reference Intakes*, 380–82.

67 Gropper, Jack L. Smith, and James L. Groff, *Advanced Nutrition and Human Metabolism*, 5th edition, Cengage Learning (2008), 114.

5

Benefits of an Early Dinner

The importance of refraining from eating a few hours before bedtime cannot be emphasized enough. In a survey of 51,529 male health professionals, it was found that late-night eating is associated with a higher BMI (obesity index), higher cholesterol levels, higher blood pressure, a higher prevalence of diabetes, and a 55 percent higher prevalence of heart disease.[68] Avoiding late-night eating is beneficial for the following reasons:

1. **Insulin resistance**: Avoiding late-night eating heals and/or prevents insulin resistance and hyperinsulinemia. Refraining from calorie intake for a few hours before bedtime enables the body's natural hormonal balance to maintain necessary energy levels by burning stored glycogen and fats. When storage space for glycogen is not full at breakfast time, the body will be more receptive to insulin and receptive to storing glycogen.[69, 70]

---

68 Leah E. Cahill et al., "Prospective Study of Breakfast Eating and Incident Coronary Heart Disease in a Cohort of Male US Health Professionals," *Circulation* (2013), vol. 128, 337–43, http://circ.ahajournals.org/content/128/4/337.full.pdf.

69 Jørgen Jensen et al., "Role of Skeletal Muscle Glycogen Breakdown for Regulation of Insulin Sensitivity by Exercise," *Frontiers in Physiology* (2011) 2: 112, http://www.ncbi.nlm.nih.gov/pmc/articles/PMC3248697/.

70 A. Zorzano et al., "Glycogen Depletion and Increased Insulin Sensitivity and Responsiveness in Muscle after Exercise," *American Journal of Physiology* 1 (December 25, 1986): 664–69, http://www.ncbi.nlm.nih.gov/pubmed/3538900.

For most people, improving insulin sensitivity is the most important reason to finish eating a few hours before bedtime. As discussed in the previous chapter, the risk of heart disease, the number one cause of death, is increased in people with insulin resistance, and it also leads to obesity and diabetes and increases the risk of contracting various cancers and other ailments.

2. **Digestion**: Avoiding late-night eating also enables the body to properly digest food and thereby avoid intestinal gases and toxins. Accumulated toxins can harm the intestines, get into the blood, and weaken the body.[71, 72]

During the sleep cycle, blood circulation and digestion slows down. There is less movement in the digestive tract (motility) and less production of digestive juices. Several digestive problems cause sleep disturbance, and, in turn, abnormal sleep brought on by these diseases is shown to contribute to the severity of these same gastrointestinal diseases and obesity.[73] The following are some of the gastrointestinal diseases that disturb sleep: gastroesophageal reflux disease (GERD), peptic ulcer, irritable bowel syndrome (IBS), and Crohn's disease (a type of inflammatory bowel disease causing a wide variety of symptoms, including abdominal pain, diarrhea, and vomiting, as well as complications outside the gastrointestinal tract such as anemia, skin rashes, arthritis, inflammation of the eye, tiredness, and lack of concentration).

---

71 R. O. Dantas and C. G. Aben-Athar, "Aspects of Sleep Effects on the Digestive Tract," *Arquivos de gastroenterologia* 1 (January–March 2002): 55–59. http://www.ncbi.nlm.nih.gov/pubmed/12184167.

72 Hye-kyung Jung, Rok Seon Choung, and Nicholas J. Talley, "Gastroesophageal Reflux Disease and Sleep Disorders: Evidence for a Causal Link and Therapeutic Implications," *Journal of Neurogastroenterology and Motility* (January 2010), http://www.ncbi.nlm.nih.gov/pmc/articles/PMC2879818/.

73 Tauseef Ali et al., "Sleep, Immunity and Inflammation in Gastrointestinal Disorders," *World Journal of Gastroenterology* (December 28, 2013), http://www.ncbi.nlm.nih.gov/pmc/articles/PMC3882397/.

During sleep, the body is in the supine position; therefore, gravity does not help the acid esophageal clearance. Additionally the primary esophageal contraction is not frequent, a fact causing a prolongation of acid clearance during sleep. Unlike digestion when sitting up, the lateral position during sleep causes more reflux episodes (acid rising from the stomach to the esophagus). The gastroesophageal reflux may be associated with nocturnal wheezing, chronic nocturnal cough, and sleep apnea (a sleep disorder characterized by pauses in breathing or instances of shallow or infrequent breathing during sleep).

A study conducted by the University of Ioannina in Greece involving five hundred healthy people found that those who had the longest interval between eating and sleeping had the lowest risk for stroke.

One theory is that the increase in acid reflux that occurs when going to sleep after a meal, combined with associated breathing impediments, contributes to causing a stroke.[74] Another theory is that the forced work of our digestive system increases blood pressure, blood sugar, and cholesterol levels, which contribute to triggering a stroke.

3. **Rest**: Avoiding late-night eating also enables the body to rest well. When the intestines are forced to digest food and the liver is forced to process elements entering the blood, blood pressure rises, preventing full and proper rest.[75] Dozens of studies link lack of rest, or short sleep, with obesity, impaired glucose tolerance, and diabetes.[76] There are also studies that demonstrate a

74 Ronnie Fass, "Sleep and Gastroesophageal Reflux Disease (GERD)," *Digestive Health Matters* 21, no. 2 (June 2012), http://www.aboutgerd.org/site/symptoms/sleep-and-gerd.

75 Hye-kyung Jung, Rok Seon Choung, and Nicholas J. Talley, "Gastroesophageal Reflux Disease and Sleep Disorders: Evidence for a Causal Link and Therapeutic Implications," *Journal of Neurogastroenterology and Motility* (January 2010), http://www.ncbi.nlm.nih.gov/pmc/articles/PMC2879818/.

76 Michael A. Grandner et al., "Problems Associated with Short Sleep: Bridging the Gap between Laboratory and Epidemiological Studies," *Sleep Medicine Reviews* (August 2010), http://www.ncbi.nlm.nih.gov/pmc/articles/PMC2888649/.

lack of sleep as a risk factor for hypertension[77] and the increased risk of developing cardiovascular diseases that comes from augmenting proinflammatory responses.[78]

4. **Secretion of Human Growth Hormone**: Avoiding late-night eating also enables the body's endocrine system to function well. The body is designed to rest at night when sleeping. During deep stages of sleep, the body secretes human growth hormone (HGH)[79] to repair and regenerate tissues, build bone and muscle, and strengthen the immune system. HGH is an outstanding beneficial hormone because it stimulates the breakdown of fat[80] while also stimulating the growth of muscle, bone, and other body fibers.[81, 82, 83] There is insufficient evidence to claim that HGH therapy can add significant muscle and strength in people who are not deficient. However, it is undisputed that deficiency leads to decreased muscle mass and exercise capacity, increased visceral fat, impaired quality of life, unfavorable alterations in lipid profile and markers of cardiovascular risk, decrease in bone mass and integrity, and increased mortality.[84]

77 J. E. Gangwisch et al., "Short Sleep Duration as a Risk Factor for Hypertension: Analyses of the First National Health and Nutrition Examination Survey," *Hypertension* (May 2006), http://www.ncbi.nlm.nih.gov/pubmed/16585410.

78 W. M. van Leeuwen et al., "Sleep Restriction Increases the Risk of Developing Cardiovascular Diseases by Augmenting Pro-Inflammatory Responses through Il-17 and CRP," *PLoS ONE* (2009), http://www.ncbi.nlm.nih.gov/pmc/articles/PMC2643002/.

79 Y. Takahashi, D. M. Kipnis, and W. H. Daughaday, "Growth Hormone Secretion during Sleep," *Journal of Clinical Investigation* 47, no. 9 (September 1968): 2079–90, http://www.ncbi.nlm.nih.gov/pmc/articles/PMC297368/pdf/jcinvest00244-0147.pdf.

80 Katarina T. Borer, "Advanced Exercise Endocrinology," *Human Kinetics* (2013): 109, 185.

81 Mary L. Reed, George R. Merriam, and Atil Y. Kargi, "Adult Growth Hormone Deficiency: Benefits, Side Effects, and Risks of Growth Hormone Replacement," *Frontiers in Endocrinology* (2013), http://www.ncbi.nlm.nih.gov/pmc/articles/PMC3671347/.

82 "Growth Hormone, Athletic Performance, and Aging," Harvard Health Publications (May 2010), http://www.health.harvard.edu/newsletters/Harvard_Mens_Health_Watch/2010/May/growth-hormone-athletic-performance-and-aging.

83 Borer, "Advanced Exercise Endocrinology," 186.

84 Reed, Merriam, and Kargi, "Adult Growth Hormone Deficiency."

Eating shortly before bedtime minimizes the secretion of HGH via *two* avenues: first, HGH is released during deep sleep—the amount of HGH secreted correlating with how much slow wave sleep (SWS) you get[85]—and since digesting food disturbs sleep inhibiting SWS, it minimizes the secretion of HGH. Second, insulin inhibits the release of HGH[86, 87] and also stifles the effectiveness of whatever HGH is released.[88] Therefore, if the late-night eating includes carbohydrates, it will cause the release of insulin, inhibiting HGH. Additionally, because one's heart rate is slower at night, the body needs to secrete more insulin than it would by day to be effective in lowering blood sugar via the transfer of glucose from the blood to the liver and muscles.

5. **Cleansing from toxins**: Fasting enables the body to cleanse itself of toxins. The longer one's daily fast period, the more effective the cleanse. (To learn more about the benefits of intermittent fasting, see chapter 9: "Daily Intermittent Fasting").

6. **Controlling calories**: Restricting one's diet by using time constraints is an effective method of lowering total daily caloric intake. Of all the times of day to restrict caloric intake, the hours before bedtime are the most important for all the above reasons. Additionally, at other times of the day, you need to digest calories in order to function your best. However, before resting at night, there is no necessity for carbohydrate loading; it is counterproductive, as already mentioned.

---

85   E. van Cauter and L. Plat, "Physiology of Growth Hormone Secretion during Sleep," *Journal of Pediatrics* (1996), http://www.ncbi.nlm.nih.gov/pubmed/8627466.

86   R. Lanzi et al., "Elevated Insulin Levels Contribute to the Reduced Growth Hormone (GH) Response to GH-Releasing Hormone in Obese Subjects," *Metabolism* (1999), http://www.ncbi.nlm.nih.gov/pubmed/10484056.

87   Hiroo Imura et al., "Effect of Adrenergic-Blocking or -Stimulating Agents on Plasma Growth Hormone, Immunoreactive Insulin, and Blood Free Fatty Acid Levels in Man," *Journal of Clinical Investigation* 50, no. 5 (May 1971), http://www.jci.org/articles/view/106578.

88   Shaonin Ji et al., "Insulin Inhibits Growth Hormone Signaling via the Growth Hormone Receptor/JAK2/STAT5B Pathway," *Journal of Biological Chemistry* (May 7, 1999), http://www.jbc.org/content/274/19/13434.full.

For those who are accustomed to eating plenty of food right up until bedtime, making an abrupt change to finishing eating two hours before bedtime will cause a problem with too much ghrelin, the hunger hormone. However, that is only a minor concern because it is only temporary. The ghrelin will stop being secreted once the body has adapted to the new eating schedule. The major difficulty, however, is *habituating* oneself to that change.

Typically, making such an abrupt change will be too challenging for most people. In all likelihood, when attempting to eat the last meal of the day so much earlier than the body is habituated to, hunger pangs will become uncontrollable shortly before bedtime.

Therefore, for most people, the most successful route of change is gradual. After getting used to a bigger interval between eating and sleeping, you can add on another twenty to thirty minutes, until the bigger interval becomes a comfortable habit. Then you can increase the interval further, and with such a gradual method of change, you can eventually become accustomed to intervals of three to four hours between eating and sleeping.

Another helpful tip is to occasionally satisfy yourself with a light piece of fruit if you realize that the increased interval is going to set your hunger out of control. That is preferable to eating other foods before sleep that create heavy workloads on the digestive system and the liver, interfering with a restful sleep.

CONCLUSION

Gradually adapt to the habit of avoiding or at least minimizing food consumption within three to four hours before bedtime to benefit from better rest, digestion, insulin sensitivity, hormonal balance, cleansing of toxins, and controlling caloric intake.

6

Exercise: The Benefits, How and When, and Making It Easy

Chapter 4 introduced Maimonides's method of curing the metabolic syndrome, including four primary elements: early dinner, exercise, late breakfast, and measured glycemic load. Maimonides's main point concerning exercise is to exert oneself sufficiently so that the body gets heated before having a meal. This improves digestion, and we know today that it also improves insulin sensitivity.

There are many factors that make exercise easier and more effective. As a certified trainer and CEO of Maimonides Health and Fitness Center, I'm proud to share my experience presenting numerous details concerning making exercise as beneficial as possible. These include:

- The Numerous Benefits of Exercise
- Why to Exercise before Meals (Especially Breakfast)
- Unique Benefits of Exercising Before Breakfast
- Aerobic or Anaerobic: Which Is Better?
- Why You Should Do Aerobic Training before Breakfast and Anaerobic Training in the Late Afternoon
- What Type of Aerobic Exercise Is the Best?
- How Much Time Should You Work Out?
- What Intensity Is Recommended?
- Is It Okay to Eat or Drink Something Before Your Prebreakfast Aerobic Workout?

- BCAA: What It Is and Why It Is So Important to Utilize When Following the Maimonides Extended Daily Intermittent Fasts
- Importance of Avoiding Muscle Breakdown after a Full-Night Fast
- Sources of BCAA: Natural and Synthetic
- Glutamine Supplementation before Breakfast
- Making Exercise Quick and Easy
- The Importance of Avoiding Prolonged Sitting

THE NUMEROUS BENEFITS OF EXERCISE

The modern world has made us less physically active than our ancestors. Considering that Maimonides prescribed physical exertion for health maintenance in his day nearly nine hundred years ago, it is even more necessary to engage in physical exertion in today's sedentary lives. Exercise is a primary element in curing us from the metabolic syndrome, and its benefits are many:

1. **Increases insulin sensitivity**: Exercising before eating meals that include carbohydrates moderates insulin secretion and enables the smaller amounts of insulin to more quickly transfer the excess blood sugar into the liver and muscles.[89]
2. **Reduces fat**: With faster insulin response and less insulin secretion, less sugar will be transformed into and stored as fat.
3. **Stabilizes blood sugar levels**: Without exercise, eating carbohydrates leads to sugar highs and then lows, followed by feelings of weakness and hunger. That roller coaster ride leads to hyperinsulinemia and obesity.
4. **Prevents disease**: Hyperinsulinemia leads to the metabolic syndrome, which leads to type 2 diabetes and heart disease. Exercising

---

89 Jørgen Jørgen Jensen et al., "Role of Skeletal Muscle Glycogen Breakdown for Regulation of Insulin Sensitivity by Exercise," *Frontiers in Physiology* (2011) 2: 112, http://www.ncbi.nlm.nih.gov/pmc/articles/PMC3248697/.

and eating at the proper times can prevent this and heal us from these illnesses.[90] According to the Institute of Medicine, it is theorized that exercise helps to protect us from cancer.[91]

5. **Strengthens heart**: Aerobic exercise strengthens the heart and cardiovascular system, adds flexibility to the blood vessels, expands the blood vessels, lowers cholesterol, and reduces high blood pressure.

6. **Increases vitality**: The intensified blood flow vitalizes all parts of the body by bringing oxygen and nutrients and removing toxins—even when you are not exercising.

7. **Improves concentration and memory**: Aerobic exercise improves concentration by increasing production of cells in the hippocampus that are responsible for memory and learning, increasing connections between brain cells, and increasing blood and oxygen to the brain.[92, 93]

8. **Prevents illness**: A stronger body is less susceptible to illnesses such as the common cold or infections.

9. **Improves hormonal balance**: Resistance training (weight lifting) boosts the production and release of beneficial hormones such as testosterone and human growth hormone—hormones that burn fat and build muscle—up to forty-eight hours after exercising. These hormones are abundant in our youth and produced and released minimally beyond middle age. Resistance training increases these hormones and their beneficial effects,

---

90   Frank B. Hu et al., "Diet, Lifestyle, and the Risk of Type 2 Diabetes Mellitus in Women," *New England Journal of Medicine* (2001), http://www.nejm.org/doi/full/10.1056/NEJMoa010492.

91   Institute of Medicine, *Dietary Reference Intakes*, 54.

92   C. Hertzog et al., "Enrichment Effects on Adult Cognitive Development: Can the Functional Capacity of Older Adults Be Preserved and Enhanced?" *Psychological Science in the Public Interest* (2008), http://www.psychologicalscience.org/journals/pspi/pdf/PSPI_9_1%20main_text.pdf.

93   Kirk I. Erickson et al., "Exercise Training Increases Size of Hippocampus and Improves Memory," Proceedings of the National Academy of Sciences USA (February 15, 2011), http://www.ncbi.nlm.nih.gov/pmc/articles/PMC3041121/

reversing the ill effects of the metabolic syndrome and restoring our vitality.[94]

10. **Improves mood**: Exercise stimulates various chemicals in the brain that improve our mood.[95, 96, 97, 98]

11. **Increases energy**: Exercise boosts our energy levels and endurance.

12. **Improves sleep**: Moderate amounts of exercise improve the quality of sleep.[99, 100]

13. **Reduces risk of injury**: Exercise improves balance and coordination, reducing the risk of falling.

14. **Strengthens bones**: Exercise maintains bone strength and protects us from osteoporosis.[101, 102]

---

94   Bente K. Pedersen and Mark A. Febbraio, "Muscles, Exercise and Obesity: Skeletal Muscle as a Secretory Organ," *Nature Reviews Endocrinology* (2012), http://www.nature.com/nrendo/journal/v8/n8/full/nrendo.2012.49.html

95   V. J. Harber and J. R. Sutton, "Endorphins and Exercise," *Sports Medicine* (1984), http://www.ncbi.nlm.nih.gov/pubmed/6091217.

96   M. Hamer, E. Stamatakis, and A. Steptoe, "Dose-Response Relationship between Physical Activity and Mental Health: The Scottish Health Survey," *British Journal of Sports Medicine* (2009), http://www.ncbi.nlm.nih.gov/pubmed/18403415

97   W. J. Strawbridge et al., "Physical Activity Reduces the Risk of Subsequent Depression for Older Adults," *American Journal of Epidemiology* 1 (2002), http://www.ncbi.nlm.nih.gov/pubmed/12181102.

98   P. B Sparling et al., "Exercise Activates the Endocannabinoid System," *Neuroreport* 14, no. 17: 2209–211, (December 2003), http://journals.lww.com/neuroreport/Abstract/2003/12020/Exercise_activates_the_endocannabinoid_system.15.aspx.

99   P. M. Buman and A. C. King, "Exercise as a Treatment to Enhance Sleep," *American Journal of Lifestyle Medicine* (November/December 2010), http://ajl.sagepub.com/content/4/6/500.abstract.

100   S. D. Youngstedt, "Effects of Exercise on Sleep," *Clinics in Sports Medicine* (2005), http://www.ncbi.nlm.nih.gov/pubmed/15892929.

101   J. J. Body et al., "Non-Pharmacological Management of Osteoporosis: A Consensus of the Belgian Bone Club," *Osteoporosis International* (November 2011), http://www.ncbi.nlm.nih.gov/pmc/articles/PMC3186889/.

102   D. Bonaiuti et al., "Exercise for Preventing and Treating Osteoporosis in Postmenopausal Women," *Cochrane Database of Systematic Reviews* (2002), http://www.ncbi.nlm.nih.gov/pubmed/12137611.

15. **Relieves stress**: Exercise reverses the detrimental effects of stress.
16. **Inspires**: Exercising inspires others to exercise.

WHY TO EXERCISE BEFORE MEALS (ESPECIALLY BREAKFAST)

There are at least three benefits of exercising before a meal that are specifically beneficial in relation to the meal:

1. **Improves digestion**: During digestion, the body produces enzymes to break down the food into smaller pieces. The nutrients derived from food are absorbed in the intestines and into the bloodstream. The blood then flows throughout the body, spreading the nutrients. As the blood circulates, the toxins are brought to the kidneys for elimination, while carbon dioxide is sent to the lungs to be exhaled.

   Both the digestive and cardiovascular systems work hard when the body has to process a lot of food. The digestive system needs more blood to do its job; therefore, blood vessels in the vicinity of the digestive system and liver expand in preparation for this. Digestive organs stimulate the heart through nerve impulses, sending signals for increased amount of blood. The heart responds accordingly by sending more blood supply to the digestive system.[103]

   Exercise gets the heart pumping hard and fast and opens up the blood vessels; done just before a meal, the increased blood flow aids in the digestive process, including the elimination of wastes.

---

103   A. F. Muller et al., "The Integrated Response of the Cardiovascular System to Food," *Digestion* (1992), http://www.ncbi.nlm.nih.gov/pubmed/1459353

2. **Improves insulin sensitivity**: Muscles that are completely filled up with glycogen stores are resistant to insulin, as they have no room to absorb more glucose. After a person exercises, the stores of glycogen are depleted, and muscles are responsive to absorbing glucose from the blood.[104] A recent study demonstrates that exercising in a fasted state improves insulin sensitivity even more than exercising after fueling up.[105]

3. **Burns more fat**: The body is almost always being fueled by both stored fats and sugars. The factors that vary are which source is dominant and how dominant it is. When glycogen (sugar) stores are low, the body speeds up fat burning in attempt to prevent using up all the sugar reserves.[106] Therefore, after fasting the whole night, when glycogen stores are low, exercise speeds up fat burning to the maximum. This was demonstrated in a controlled study of twenty young male volunteers in a six-week endurance-training program comparing fat burning between those who performed the endurance training in a fasted state to those who performed after fueling up on carbohydrates. Not only did the men in the fasting state burn more fat, but their sugar levels proved more stable, and they lost more weight as well.[107]

---

104 Jørgen Jørgen Jensen et al., "Role of Skeletal Muscle Glycogen Breakdown for Regulation of Insulin Sensitivity by Exercise," *Frontiers in Physiology* (2011) 2: 112, http://www.ncbi.nlm.nih.gov/pmc/articles/PMC3248697/.

105 K. van Proeyen et al., "Training in the Fasted State Improves Glucose Tolerance during Fat-Rich Diet," *Journal of Physiology* (2010), http://www.ncbi.nlm.nih.gov/pubmed/20837645.

106 Katarina T. Borer, "Advanced Exercise Endocrinology," *Human Kinetics* (2013): 106.

107 K. van Proeyen et al., "Beneficial Metabolic Adaptations Due to Endurance Exercise Training in the Fasted State," *Journal of Applied Physiology* (2011), http://www.ncbi.nlm.nih.gov/nlmcatalog?term=%22J+Appl+Physiol+(1985)%22[Title+Abbreviation

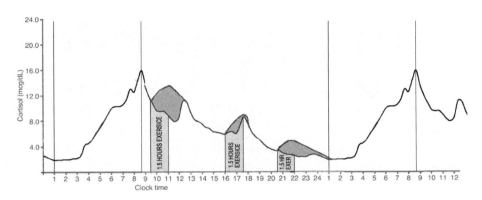

Figure 6-1. The effects of 1.5 hours exercise
on the circadian rhythm of cortisol

In respect to maximizing the fat-burning effects of exercise, it is fascinating and useful to know how to synchronize one's exercise with the circadian rhythm of one's cortisol levels, as cortisol is one of the most powerful fat-burning hormones we have. Normally, cortisol reaches its lowest daily levels around midnight, when it begins a steady climb up to the daily peak levels one half hour after waking up, at which point a decline begins, with two or three slight rises over the course of the day. Typically, the highest peak will be around 8:30 a.m. (for a person who wakes up at 8:00 a.m.), with the second highest minipeak happening around 1:30 p.m. and another one or two minipeaks at lower levels later in the afternoon, up until the early evening, when the downward trend begins to flatten out toward the midnight bottom. If you begin an exercise workout sometime in the middle of the day, if the exercise coincides with your circadian midday *rise toward* a minipeak, or if the exercise coincides with the midday minipeak, the exercise won't significantly influence his or her cortisol secretion (figure 6-1, exercising from 4:00 p.m. to 5:30 p.m.). However, if the time you exercise coincides with the time when your cortisol is on a decline or at basal level, the exercise will cause a major change by forcing cortisol to rise—going in the opposite direction of the circadian rhythm (figure 6-1, exercising from 9:30 a.m. to 11:00 a.m. or 8:30 p.m. to 10:00 p.m.). The effect can be maximized with a ninety-minute moderate-intensity aerobic exercise (between 25–55% of maximum effort), either late morning or late evening.[108] Late evening can be a problematic time to exercise if it forces you to eat late afterward or if it makes falling asleep difficult. But for those who can work exercise into their schedules before breakfast, the fat-burning effect will be the most powerful possible.

UNIQUE BENEFITS OF EXERCISING BEFORE BREAKFAST

In particular, exercising before breakfast is beneficial (more so than before other meals), as it increases blood circulation when circulation is slowest. During non-rapid-eye-movement sleep, the heart rate and blood pressure drop as breathing slows, and the core body temperature falls. Additionally, the cerebral blood flow drops, and the overall cardiac output is lowered. One of the functions of sleeping is to give the heart a chance to rest after an active day. Exercise gets the heart pumping again,

- dissipating the grogginess of sleep;
- increasing cerebral blood flow, and thereby increasing alertness of the mind; and
- increasing blood flow to the limbs and organs, giving vitality and energy.

AEROBIC OR ANAEROBIC: WHICH IS BETTER?

Anaerobic training (resistance training) focuses on building muscle and strength, whereas aerobic training focuses on strengthening the cardio-vascular system, lungs, and endurance. Both types of exercise help reduce fat. Aerobic training is more effective in the short term, as it burns calories faster; however, in the long term, adding muscle mass burns off fat in a variety of ways:

1. Resistance training causes the body to produce and release more HGH and testosterone, which builds muscle and burns fat.

---

108 Katarina T. Borer, "Advanced Exercise Endocrinology," *Human Kinetics* (2013): 211.

2. The body burns calories during the chemical and biological processes of building muscle tissue.
3. Having more muscle mass requires burning more calories to sustain that mass, even when sleeping. An added bonus to muscle mass is that, in general, the body uses fat as a source of energy for sustaining the muscles.

So building muscle and maintaining it are important for fighting obesity and consequently are important for fighting the metabolic syndrome, type 2 diabetes, and heart disease. However, for improving circulation and reducing blood pressure, aerobic exercise is more effective. It should be noted that very intensive strength training requires much food for the muscles to recuperate and rebuild between training sessions, and requires increased insulin to drive the nutrients into the muscle tissue; this can lead to fat gain as well. In general, for most people, doctors recommend performing both types of exercise—aerobic and resistance.

So instead of asking which type of exercise is better, the question we should ask is what the most advantageous time of day is for each type of exercise.

Ideally, aerobic exercise should be done in the morning before breakfast, and resistance training should be done in the late afternoon.

WHY YOU SHOULD DO AEROBIC TRAINING BEFORE BREAKFAST AND ANAEROBIC TRAINING IN THE LATE AFTERNOON

Hormonal Response

In the morning, cortisol levels are at their peak (cortisol levels reach lowest levels at around midnight; levels start to rise at around 2:00 a.m. to 3:00 a.m. and reach a peak at around 8:30 a.m. for a person who wakes up at 8:00 a.m.). Cortisol levels then slowly decrease back to the nadir to complete the twenty-four hour cycle. The peak cortisol level is approximately 399 nmol/l, whilst the nadir is <50 nmol/l.[109]

Cortisol is a catabolic hormone. Cortisol provides energy by breaking down fats and proteins (including muscle fiber, when alternative sources are depleted) when fasting throughout the night. Therefore, attempting to build muscle with resistance training would be somewhat counterproductive in the morning—the time when cortisol is most actively breaking down protein. Resistance training actually weakens the muscles temporarily during the workout (try to continue lifting your maximum weight after having already exhausted yourself). Resistance training strengthens the muscles via *recovery* from the workout, which can take forty-eight hours or more.

Resistance (Muscle Building) Training Is Best in Late Afternoon

Resistance training can be performed at times other than the ideal time of late afternoon, but should never be done on an empty stomach after an all-night fast. When done in the late afternoon, at least two hours after a hearty meal, you experience:

1. **Less cortisol**: In the afternoon, there is less cortisol to interfere with recovery as explained here: "Optimal adaptations to resistance training (i.e., muscle hypertrophy and strength increases) occur when an athlete performs training in the late afternoon. At that time, exercise-induced increases in testosterone concentration coincide with a circadian *decline* in concentrations of the catabolic hormone cortisol."[110]

2. **A greater anabolic response**: The body's response to producing and releasing testosterone is greater in the late afternoon, enhancing quicker and more potent recovery and building of

---

109 Sharon Chan and Miguel Debono, "Replication of Cortisol Circadian Rhythm: New Advances in Hydrocortisone Replacement Therapy," *Therapeutic Advances in Endocrinology and Metabolism* (June 2010), http://www.ncbi.nlm.nih.gov/pmc/articles/PMC3475279/.
110 Katarina T. Borer, "Advanced Exercise Endocrinology," *Human Kinetics* (2013): 215.

muscle, as explained here: "Although testosterone levels are higher in the morning, an increased resistance exercise-induced testosterone response has been found in the late afternoon, suggesting greater responsiveness of the hypothalamo-pituitary-testicular axis then."[111]

Aerobic (Fat Burning Plus Endurance) Training Is Best before Breakfast

Based on the body's hormonal status before breakfast, aerobic exercise is more advantageous than resistance training in the morning for the following reasons:

1. **It is not in conflict with cortisol.** Aerobic training burns calories faster than anaerobic training, but it does not tax the muscles or break down muscle fiber as much as resistance training.

2. **It is the best time for fat burning.** When the body burns calories through exercise, a percentage of those calories come from glycogen stores in the liver and muscles, and a percentage come from fats that are broken down and consumed. Aerobic exercise burns fat faster than resistance training. The body burns fat faster when glycogen reserves are lower than when they are full,[112] so the longer the aerobic workout, the lower glycogen reserves get, and the faster the body burns fat. Performing aerobics in the morning burns fat faster than at other times of the day for at least two reasons: first, glycogen reserves are at their lowest, and second, the fat burning hormone cortisol is at its peak. So prior to breakfast is the worst time for resistance training, as it would break down muscle and delay recovery, but it is

---

111 L. D. Hayes, G. F. Bickerstaff, and J. S. Baker, "Interactions of Cortisol, Testosterone, and Resistance Training: Influence of Circadian Rhythms," *Chronobiology International* (June 2010), http://www.ncbi.nlm.nih.gov/pubmed/20560706.

112 Katarina T. Borer, "Advanced Exercise Endocrinology," *Human Kinetics* (2013): 106.

the best time for fat-burning-aerobics, as it is the most effective time for using aerobics to burn fat.

3. **It helps you wake up and become alert.** Aerobic training directly increases blood circulation, and as such it is more effective than anaerobic training in getting the body out of the sleep mode.

4. **It improves insulin sensitivity.** Aerobics burn calories faster, and as such it is more effective in the short term for improving insulin sensitivity. It is the most effective way to avoid the hyperinsulinemic response to breakfast.

WHAT TYPE OF AEROBIC EXERCISE IS THE BEST?

Ideally, you should choose exercise equipment and/or a place that is the most conducive for you personally to do the exercise nearly every day before breakfast. Based on one's time and budget constraints as well as physical limitations, each individual has different needs. Some people are bored exercising indoors, while others won't maintain an outdoor exercise schedule that is disrupted by weather interferences such as rain, heat, cold, and so on. Some people need the atmosphere of a gym to get them going; others can stick to an exercise schedule at home, but getting out to the gym takes too much time and effort to maintain.

The best aerobic exercise is the one that you as an individual are most likely to perform regularly in the long term.

Here are some options that don't require any equipment:

- Walking or running
- Running in place
- Jumping jacks
- Dancing
- Walking up flights of stairs

And here are options that require equipment:

- Jumping rope
- Roller-skating
- Regular or stationary biking
- Elliptical training
- Indoor or outdoor rowing
- Punching bags
- Treadmills
- Electric stair climbers

HOW MUCH TIME SHOULD YOU WORK OUT?

In general, more is better, so long as you don't overstrain yourself. The longer the session, the faster the fat burning becomes (because as the glycogen reserves become depleted, the body relies more on stored fat as the source of energy). When plasma-glucose concentrations decrease below the regulated range, secretion of glucagon, cortisol, adrenaline, and growth hormone are triggered, releasing fatty acids from storage into the blood for fuel. Additionally, when glycogen is depleted from liver stores, gluconeogenesis is activated, which is the process generating the conversion of proteins and fats into glucose, and lipolysis is activated, which is the process of releasing fat stores into circulation to be burned directly as fuel,[113] thus speeding up and maximizing fat loss. And, of course, the longer the workout, the more you will improve your cardiovascular condition (assuming you don't overtrain—you shouldn't exercise so much that the length of the recuperation would prevent further progress).

Concerning exercise, anything is better than nothing. Even a small amount can bring a significant improvement in insulin sensitivity. *The main focus should be keeping the frequency to more than three days a week and ideally daily.* The secondary focus should be striving to attain linear progress increasing the length and intensity of the workouts as one's abilities improve.

---

113   Katarina T. Borer, "Advanced Exercise Endocrinology," *Human Kinetics* (2013): 105–110.

WHAT INTENSITY IS RECOMMENDED?

Beginners should start out at low intensity but strive to improve their physical condition by increasing the intensity as their condition improves. There is a trade-off between intensity and endurance. The greater the intensity of the workout, the more limited one's ability to endure extending the length of the workout. For beginners, it is usually advisable to focus more on endurance than intensity. Additionally, for the purpose of burning fat and improving insulin sensitivity, endurance workouts are more effective, as the extended time burns more calories in total. But if you can do aerobics for more than forty minutes, consider increasing the intensity and/or incorporating "interval training." Interval training is changing the intensity for intervals of time or distance. For example, you could walk up three flights of stairs slowly and then one flight quickly, three flights slowly and one quickly. Or you could combine short spurts of running fast with intervals of walking or jogging for a minute or two.

If you incorporate resistance training in the afternoons, you should go light on the intensity of the aerobic workout in the morning beforehand so that you can apply maximum intensity during the resistance training.

IS IT OKAY TO EAT OR DRINK SOMETHING BEFORE YOUR PREBREAKFAST AEROBIC WORKOUT?

Water is necessary, so obviously there are no limitations on that. Beverages with caffeine that don't have sugar or protein (milk has both protein and sugar) are fine in moderation. Actually, there are varying opinions concerning the pros and cons of caffeine—it does speed up metabolism, but the catabolic effects can inhibit muscle development.

Having a prebreakfast snack (less than the size of one mouthful—the equivalent of the volume of an egg),[114] consisting of small quan-

---

114 Rashi's commentary of Talmud tractate Succah page 26A: "A snack as was customary to taste food (the volume of one mouthful) on the way to the study hall."

tity of fruit or vegetable and/or a small portion of protein, one and a half to two hours after waking up, is 100 percent acceptable and even recommended by the Talmud.[115] Since cortisol begins to decline from its peak half an hour after waking up, it won't be so high 1.5–2 hours after waking up, and such a snack with few carbohydrates and no major protein intake will not invoke much of an insulin response. Therefore, the dangerous conflict of cortisol and insulin opposing each other won't occur. The advantage of the snack is to avoid using body proteins for fuel, as one's glycogen reserves are low after fasting all night, forcing the body to increase the use of other stored energy. Keep in mind, however, that although amino acids (proteins) do not invoke as strong an insulin response as carbohydrates, they do, however, invoke an insulin response.[116] Therefore, the closer in time you are to your cortisol peak (half an hour after waking up), the more careful you need to be to avoid a surge of insulin. So, if you're having a prebreakfast protein snack, it still needs to be small (eighty to one hundred calories total) and not eaten too early.

A drink with added powered BCAA is customarily ingested by athletes before workouts. But even for nonathletes, if you are planning to work out after having fasted more than ten hours, BCAA can be a great health boost.

BCAA: WHAT IT IS AND WHY IT IS SO IMPORTANT TO UTILIZE WHEN FOLLOWING THE MAIMONIDES EXTENDED DAILY INTERMITTENT FASTS

BCAAs, or branched chain amino acids, are three amino acids: leucine, isoleucine, and valine. BCAAs are among the nine essential amino acids for humans, accounting for 35 percent of the essential amino acids in muscle tissue proteins.

---

115 Talmud tractate Succah page 26A: "A snack as was customary to taste food (the volume of one mouthful) on the way to the study hall." The Tur in ch. 155 of Ohr HaChaim writes that it is recommended to have such a snack.

116 McClenaghan et al., "Amino Acid–Induced Insulin Secretion."

BCAAs are unique compared to all the seventeen other amino acids in that they can be oxidized (burned) in the muscle as fuel. As such, during intensive or prolonged exercise, the BCAAs inside the muscle are used as fuel and become depleted in the muscle tissue. Digesting proteins high in BCAAs just before a workout would theoretically protect the muscle from depletion of BCAAs; however, shortly before exercising, it is counterproductive to digest anything that needs to be processed by the liver, because when the liver works, it deprives the muscles of blood flow and energy. Additionally, the exercise impedes the simultaneous digestion of food and the ability of the liver to process the food. Since BCAAs are "free-form" amino acids as opposed to bonded amino acids in long chains of complete proteins, they don't need to be broken down and processed further by the liver. Rather, they bypass the liver, going straight into the blood, absorbed quickly by the muscles. Therefore, they can be ingested immediately before and even during workouts and are commonly utilized by athletes to

1. improve exercise performance,
2. reduce muscle-protein breakdown during intense exercise,
3. speed recovery and rebuilding of muscle after exercise,
4. curb appetite, and
5. minimize immune suppression resulting from exercise.

IMPORTANCE OF AVOIDING MUSCLE BREAKDOWN AFTER A FULL-NIGHT FAST

Exercising always places a toll on energy reserves and depletes the liver of glycogen, thereby activating gluconeogenesis—the conversion of fat and protein into glucose.[117] In the morning, when the catabolic hormone cortisol is at its peak, the body is already getting most of its glucose via gluconeogenesis, as that is one of the functions of cortisol.

When following the Maimonides-prescribed extended daily fast (chapter 9), keep in mind that in the morning, after ten or more hours

---

117 Katarina T. Borer, "Advanced Exercise Endocrinology," *Human Kinetics* (2013): 107.

of fasting, glycogen reserves are low, and the body aims to maximize burning fats (lipolysis) and converting proteins and fat to glucose for fuel (gluconeogenesis). It does this to maintain homeostasis and preserve the remaining glycogen reserves.

In summary, when following the Maimonides method of diet and exercise, three factors combine to intensify the metabolic process of gluconeogenesis:

1. Low glycogen reserves from fasting
2. Peak cortisol levels
3. Energy needs for exercise

That's great for burning fat but a serious concern for muscle loss, since the body also burns muscle as fuel when gluconeogenesis gets intense.

Digesting BCAAs protects the muscles from being used as fuel while providing energy without raising blood sugar levels or insulin. And without the infringement of insulin, BCAA consumption enables continued burning of fats for fuel, in contrast to carbohydrate consumption, which inhibits the burning of fats by causing the body to release insulin. So it is highly recommended to have about five grams of BCAA per half hour of exercise; be sure to mix it with sufficient water to avoid dehydration, as the muscles absorb water together with the BCAA. Sixteen ounces of water is recommended for five grams of BCAA.

The bottom line before breakfast:

BCAA enables burning fat and preserving muscle!

SOURCES OF BCAA: NATURAL AND SYNTHETIC

Proteins are large biological molecules consisting of one or more long chains of amino acids linked by peptide bonds; however, most sources of protein don't have all twenty amino acids. Meat, fish, dairy, and eggs have all the essential amino acids, including the three branched-chain amino acids. Soy also has BCAAs in lesser concentration.

However, BCAAs in pure form—separate from mixture with other amino acids, dietary fiber, carbohydrates, or fats and without the peptide bonds that combine them into long chains—are only available on the market in the form produced in laboratories from sugar. Similar to the process of wine making, in which sugar is fermented by yeast with the chemical reaction yielding alcohol, BCAAs are manufactured by fermenting sugar with particular cultures that yield certain amino acids. Once converted to BCAAs, they contain no remnants of sugar.

Complete proteins, which are made up of long chains of amino acids, place a toll on the digestive system and the processing that takes place in the liver and therefore should preferably not be consumed in significant quantities shortly before or during exercise. But laboratory-produced BCAAs are absorbed immediately into the blood and into the muscles and therefore can be used shortly before and during exercise. It is highly recommended that they be taken in the morning when following the Maimonides prescription of exercising after a long fast of early dinner and before a late breakfast. Doing so energizes you for your prebreakfast workout and protects you from burning muscle tissue for fuel, yet it doesn't raise sugar or insulin levels.

GLUTAMINE SUPPLEMENTATION BEFORE BREAKFAST

Glutamine is the most abundant amino acid in muscle and blood plasma. It is considered to be a nonessential amino acid because it is made by the body and is not absolutely required to be obtained through the diet. Although we do get glutamine in our diets, it is necessary for the body to produce more to meet the vast amounts required.

Glutamine has many functions, one of which is being used for fuel in gluconeogenesis, the process of the body creating glucose from stored fats and proteins.

If you are on a low-carbohydrate diet, exercise a lot, and burn more calories than you take in, your body creates the glucose it needs from fats and from the amino acids alanine and glutamine during the metabolic process called gluconeogenesis. If you do this day after day, glutamine reserves in the muscles can fall so low that muscle tissue is consumed for energy needs. Therefore, for people on weight-loss diets or who exercise intensely on a routine basis, taking glutamine supplementation can help maintain muscle mass and even enable the body to build muscle despite taking in fewer calories than are burned.

The more a person works out in an effort to enhance muscle growth, the more glutamine is used and the greater the immediate catabolic response (breaking down fats and proteins as opposed to anabolic building). Since glutamine is a primary source of fuel for the cells of the immune system, depleting it not only weakens the muscles, but it also makes one more susceptible to disease and infections as a result of lowered immunity.

Individuals digesting sufficient proteins a few times a day, especially after workouts, may not need supplementation of glutamine; however, in the morning, when exercising before breakfast, one's body is in an intense catabolic state. To prevent the consumption of glutamine in muscle, you can supplement with five grams of glutamine. Since it is an amino acid as opposed to a protein (a chain of amino acids), digesting it will not tax the body or interfere with the workout.

A total of ten to twenty-five grams of amino acids (glutamine and BCAAs) could be a sufficient intake for muscle preservation, but they're not a significant enough amount to be considered a meal, and with zero carbs, you still get virtually all the benefits of the prolonged daily intermittent fasting.

MAKING EXERCISE QUICK AND EASY

Making exercise quick, easy, appealing, and convenient is the key to being able to adhere to a daily program for life. Ideally we need to do aerobic exercise daily or at least three times a week. Also ideally, the aerobics should be done before breakfast. If you habituate yourself to exercise even for as little as three to four minutes daily—every day—eventually it becomes easier to accustom yourself to longer sessions. Some people start out attempting long and hard workouts, thinking that anything less is not significant. However, many people can become discouraged that they are not living up to their plans, and the risk of discarding the whole program is greater than most people realize. The value of just getting the blood circulating and body warmed up with a few minutes of exercise before a meal cannot be overestimated; when performed daily, the difference it makes on one's health is the difference between day and night.

THE IMPORTANCE OF AVOIDING PROLONGED SITTING

According to a fourteen-year study of over 120,000 adults[118] and a twelve-year study of 17,000 adults,[119] prolonged sitting is associated with cardiovascular disease and mortality. A reduction in time spent sitting demonstrates significant health benefits.

Furthermore, a controlled study of 168 adults for seven days revealed that independent of total sedentary time and moderate-to-vigorous intensity of activity, increased breaks in sedentary time are beneficially associated with waist circumference, BMI, triglycerides, and 2-h plasma glucose.[120]

In other words, make a point of getting on your feet often throughout the day, and break long periods of sitting as often as possible. This alone has significant health benefits.

---

118   A. V. Patel et al., "Leisure Time Spent Sitting in Relation to Total Mortality in a Prospective Cohort of US Adults." *American Journal of Epidemiology* (2010), http://www.ncbi.nlm.nih.gov/pubmed/20650954.

119   N. Owen, A. Bauman, and W. Brown, "Too Much Sitting: A Novel and Important Predictor of Chronic Disease Risk?" *Medicine and Science in Sports and Exercise* (2009), http://www.ncbi.nlm.nih.gov/pubmed/19346988.

120   G. N. Healy et al., "Breaks in Sedentary Time: Beneficial Associations with Metabolic Risk," *Diabetes Care* (2008), http://www.ncbi.nlm.nih.gov/pubmed/18252901.

CONCLUSION

1. Aerobics are most effective before breakfast.
2. Anaerobic exercises should never be done before breakfast and are most effective in the late afternoon.
3. Strive to exercise every day, even if it's just a little. Progress first by extending the length of the sessions, and then by increasing the intensity.
4. BCAAs and glutamine are helpful prebreakfast and preworkout supplements.
5. Avoid sitting for prolonged periods; break up the time with walking or standing.

7

Late Breakfast: When, Why, and What to Eat

A late breakfast is the third of the four primary elements that cure and shield us from the metabolic syndrome. As I explained, hyperinsulinemia is the root cause of the metabolic syndrome. Cortisol is an antagonist to insulin, and eating breakfast early, when cortisol levels are highest, will exacerbate hyperinsulinemia. Whereas insulin acts to lower blood sugar levels, cortisol does just the opposite and raises them. Whereas insulin acts to direct fat metabolism toward storage, cortisol releases stored fats, directing metabolism toward fuel consumption. This chapter explains the following:

- Morning Cortisol Levels
- The Drawbacks of Eating Breakfast Too Early
- The Drawbacks of Eating Breakfast Too Late
- The Ideal Time for Breakfast
- Are There Scientific Studies That Dispute the Recommendation of the Talmud to Eat Breakfast as Late as Six Hours after Awakening?
- What to Eat for Breakfast
- Making Sure the Carbohydrates Are Absorbed Slowly
- A Balanced Breakfast
- Summary
- Appendix: Late Breakfast: The Moral Significance According to the Talmud

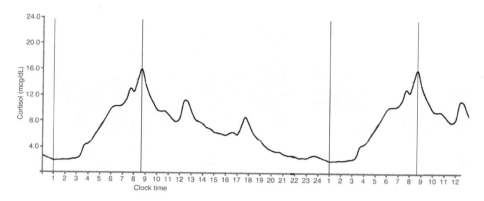

Figure 7-1. Fluctuations in cortisol levels around the clock

MORNING CORTISOL LEVELS

While affected slightly by stress and blood sugar levels, cortisol blood levels are dictated primarily by a circadian rhythm. As previously described, this typically reaches a low point around midnight. Around 2:00 a.m. it begins a steep climb upward to its pinnacle at 8:30 a.m. (for a person who wakes up at 8:00 a.m.). It then turns downward again until midnight, with one to three slight turns upward over the course of the day, most notably at midday (figure 7-1). Peak cortisol blood concentration after waking up is about eight times the concentration that it is at the daily low point.[121]

Rising nighttime cortisol levels ensure sufficient blood sugar levels over the course of the night. Another reason the body secretes more and more cortisol as wake-up time approaches is to give us the energy to wake up from sleep mode. Furthermore, waking up stimulates ACTH (adrenocorticotropic hormone) secretion in the pituitary gland, which then stimulates cortisol secretion in the adrenal glands. This additional boost of cortisol after waking up energizes us for physical activity at the start of our day despite a lengthy fasted state. Physiologists refer to

---

121 Sharon Chan and Miguel Debono, "Replication of Cortisol Circadian Rhythm: New Advances in Hydrocortisone Replacement Therapy," *Therapeutic Advances in Endocrinology and Metabolism* (June 2010), http://www.ncbi.nlm.nih.gov/pmc/articles/PMC3475279/.

this rapid increase and peak in cortisol level after waking up as *cortisol awakening response*, or CAR.

High cortisol levels in the morning explain why many people are not hungry at this point of the day, since cortisol raises blood sugar levels, sufficing our energy needs. Hunger upon waking up is often because of habituation to an early breakfast, which sets a timer for the release of gastric acids and the hormone ghrelin, making us hungry. However, the high cortisol levels ensure sufficient blood sugar levels to carry on physical activities for at least a few hours before necessitating ingesting the first meal of the day.

THE DRAWBACKS OF EATING BREAKFAST TOO EARLY

As mentioned, cortisol is the antagonist of insulin—whereas insulin lowers blood sugar levels, cortisol raises them. If breakfast is eaten when cortisol levels are at their highest, the insulin that is secreted in response to the raised sugar levels from breakfast will be ineffective due to the countereffects of the cortisol. That is insulin resistance. To lower the blood sugar levels to a healthy level, the body will then be forced to release huge amounts of insulin. This theory is supported by research finding that insulin response to a meal is higher in the morning than in the afternoon.[122] Inevitably, blood sugar levels will drop after the meal. When they drop too low, the body releases hormones such as adrenaline, glucagon, and cortisol to raise them back up. However, due to the extremely high levels of insulin that were released just a short time earlier and still remain (insulin goes through a process of degradation that takes about an hour after a meal is eaten in healthy individuals;[123] and in people with hyperinsulinemia, the

---

122 Daniela Jakubowicz et al., "Differential Morning vs. Evening Insulin and Glucagon-Like Peptide-1 (GLP-1) Responses after Identical Meal in Type 2 Diabetic Subjects," *Endocrine Society* (June 2014), http://press.endocrine.org/doi/abs/10.1210/endo-meetings.2014.DGM.16.SUN-1058.

123 William C. William C. Duckworth, Robert G. Bennett, and Frederick G. Hamel, "Insulin Degradation: Progress and Potential," *Endocrine Reviews* (July 1, 2013), http://press.endocrine.org/doi/full/10.1210/edrv.19.5.0349.

process of insulin clearance is impaired, extending the process for a longer time[124]), these blood sugar–raising hormones will not be effective. This explains why people get sugar lows and hunger pains just an hour or two after eating a hearty breakfast "too early" (at a time when cortisol levels are high and the body is resistant to insulin). If eating an early breakfast is a daily occurrence, the extreme and chronic levels of adrenaline, glucagon, and cortisol fight the high levels of insulin and become toxic and harmful to the entire body. Long-term high levels of toxicity cause numerous health risks and illnesses, including an increase in the number of fat cells,[125, 126] leading to chronic fat-mass increase (as explained in part I).

THE DRAWBACKS OF EATING BREAKFAST TOO LATE

If one eats breakfast "too late" on a daily basis, there are also negative ramifications:

1. The body decomposes muscle fiber to be used for energy.
2. The body slows down the metabolic rate to conserve energy.
3. The person experiences fatigue and less ability to concentrate and function well.
4. Since the body has many intertwined systems that operate around the biological clock, delaying breakfast "too late" on a daily basis causes these systems to get out of sync. This causes functionality to break down, leading to physical weakness and susceptibility to illness.

---

124 M. E. Valera Mora et al, "Insulin Clearance in Obesity," *Journal of the American College of Nutrition*, (December 2003), http://www.ncbi.nlm.nih.gov/pubmed/14684753.

125 H. Hauner, P. Schmid, and E. R. Pfeiffer, "Glucocorticoids and Insulin promote the differentiation of human adipocyte precursor cells into fat cells," *Journal of Clinical Endocrinology and Metabolism* (April 1987), http://www.ncbi.nlm.nih.gov/pubmed/3546356.

126 F. Grégoire, C. Genart, N. Hauser, and C. Remacle, "Glucocorticoids Induce a Drastic Inhibition of proliferation and stimulate differentiation of adult rat fat cell precursors," *Experimental Cell Research* (October 1991), http://www.ncbi.nlm.nih.gov/pubmed/1893938.

THE IDEAL TIME FOR BREAKFAST

We know that eating breakfast first thing in the morning leads to hyperinsulinemia, and delaying breakfast until very late leads to the above-mentioned harmful effects. So, what is the ideal time to eat breakfast?

According to the Talmud,[127] the ideal time to eat breakfast is three to six hours after waking. Additionally, if you have a small snack in the morning, breakfast can be delayed even past noon without suffering from any of the above-mentioned harmful effects.

ARE THERE SCIENTIFIC STUDIES THAT DISPUTE THE RECOMMENDATION OF THE TALMUD TO EAT BREAKFAST AS LATE AS SIX HOURS AFTER AWAKENING?

A sixteen-year study of nearly twenty-seven thousand men found that those who skipped breakfast had a 27 percent greater risk of chronic heart disease.[128] A ten-year study of twenty thousand men found that participants who skipped breakfast were 15 percent more likely to have substantial weight gain (≥ 5 kg) during ten years of follow-up.[129] And a sixteen-year study of twenty-nine thousand men found that participants who skipped breakfast were 21 percent more likely to develop type 2 diabetes mellitus.[130]

It would appear that these three studies propose an insurmountable challenge to our premise that eating a late breakfast is beneficial. But,

---

127 Talmud, Tractate Pesachim 12b, and Tractate Shabbas 10a, and Shulchan Aruch, Aruch Chaim, chapter 157. The Mishna Brura writes in the name of the Magen Avroham that the hours mentioned in the Talmud are calculated from the time of awakening.

128 Leah E. Cahill et al., "Prospective Study of Breakfast Eating and Incident Coronary Heart Disease in a Cohort of Male US Health Professionals," *Circulation* (2013), vol. 128, 337–43, http://circ.ahajournals.org/content/128/4/337.full.pdf.

129 Amber A. W. A. van der Heijden et al., "A Prospective Study of Breakfast Consumption and Weight Gain among US Men," *Obesity* (2007), http://onlinelibrary.wiley.com/doi/10.1038/oby.2007.292/full.

130 R. A. Mekary et al., "Eating Patterns and Type 2 Diabetes Risk in Men: Breakfast Omission, Eating Frequency, and Snacking," *American Journal of Clinical Nutrition* (2012), http://ajcn.nutrition.org/content/95/5/1182.full.

upon deeper investigation, it turns out that all these studies included the exact same wording in their questionnaire: "Please indicate the times of day that you usually eat (mark all that apply): before breakfast, breakfast, between breakfast and lunch, lunch, between lunch and dinner, dinner, between dinner and bed time, and after going to bed." The studies also defined *breakfast* as a positive response to any of the first three eating times (before breakfast, breakfast, and between breakfast and lunch).

Since the Talmud recommends having a light prebreakfast snack, that would qualify as "a positive response to the first eating time (before breakfast)." And even without the prebreakfast snack, eating a late breakfast would also qualify as "between breakfast and lunch," which is defined as breakfast by these studies (a positive response to any of the first three eating times). Therefore, according to the three studies quoted above, the Talmud's recommendations are categorized as a diet that doesn't skip breakfast.

There is no lack of nutritionists and studies espousing the propagandistic mantra that "skipping" breakfast has all sorts of harmful effects. What is lacking, however, are legitimate controlled studies comparing an early breakfast to a late breakfast.

There is also a major difference between the effects on a person accustomed to eating an early breakfast but skips it and a person who is accustomed to eating a late breakfast. The primary difference is the release of ghrelin, the hunger hormone released at the time you are habituated to eat. If you are habituated to eating an early breakfast but skip it, you will suffer the harms of elevated ghrelin levels (as explained in chapter 1), whereas a person habituated to a late breakfast won't have elevated ghrelin levels.

If you decide to follow the recommendation of the Talmud of waiting three to six hours for breakfast, with a small prebreakfast snack, you should *adjust gradually* to the changes over a period of as much as a few months, becoming comfortable with the gradual changes until eventually habituated in accordance with the Talmud.

WHAT TO EAT FOR BREAKFAST

It appears there is no consensus among dietitians concerning how to divide up one's planned macronutrient consumption over the course of the day. Some dietitians, like Nancy Clark, MS, RD, adhere to the proverb "Eat breakfast like a king, lunch like a prince, and dinner like a pauper." Clark and others emphasize fueling up with healthy carbohydrates for breakfast. Others, like Dr. Sears, recommend dividing meals, snacks, and macronutrients evenly throughout the day.

Specifically in regards to carbohydrates as opposed to the other macronutrients, some dietitians recommend that breakfast should include more carbohydrates than other meals in order to supply the body energy *before* doing activities. This is paralleled in Jewish law and custom, and in the biblical verse Exodus 16:8: "G-d will give you meat in the evening to eat, and bread in the morning to satisfy you." From this verse we see that in the evening, the main course should be protein, while for breakfast, the main course should be carbohydrates—energy food. This principle of having the majority of one's carbohydrates early in the day to provide the energy needed before the bulk of our activity is very logical; it should be obvious that eating a high-carbohydrate meal before becoming inactive—going to sleep for the night—is counterproductive.

If you follow the guidelines of Maimonides—finishing dinner early and eating breakfast late after doing at least a minimal amount of exercise—your storage of glycogen will be at its daily lowest in the morning. And with the whole day in front of you, breakfast is the most important time to stock up on carbohydrates to ensure that you have the energy to function your best.

In regard to the concern of high-carbohydrate meals causing high blood sugar and obesity, if you follow all of Maimonides's recommendations—*preparing the body to be highly responsive to insulin* by eating an early dinner and late breakfast, plus exercise—a healthy but reasonable portion of carbohydrates will not spike insulin too much with most people.

MAKING SURE THE CARBOHYDRATES ARE ABSORBED SLOWLY

We need to replenish our glycogen stores in the morning to maximize our abilities to function our best throughout the day. To do this in a controlled manner so that the carbohydrates are absorbed slowly and steadily, as opposed to shocking the blood with a sugar spike that quickly fizzles out to a sugar low a short time later, do the following:

1. Ensure that most of the consumed carbohydrates have a low glycemic index.
2. Balance carbohydrates with fiber, proteins, and healthy fats. These types of foods slow down the absorption of the carbohydrates into the blood, give us a feeling of satiety,[131] and additionally provide calories for energy once the sugar level eventually begins to drop. This thereby stabilizes the sugar level for more time, providing energy longer and pushing off hunger further,[132] while improving insulin sensitivity.[133]

A BALANCED BREAKFAST

Breakfast also needs to include vitamins and minerals. Whole grains, fresh fruits, and vegetables are healthy sources of carbohydrates that include plenty of fiber, vitamins, and minerals. Nuts and seeds have healthy fats and some protein as well as plenty of vitamins and minerals. Chapter 11, "Protein" explains in detail the best sources of protein and how much is needed daily, specifically for breakfast.

---

131   T. J. Little and C. Feinle-Bisset, "Effects of Dietary Fat on Appetite and Energy Intake in Health and Obesity—Oral and Gastrointestinal Sensory Contributions," *Physiology and Behavior* (2011), http://www.ncbi.nlm.nih.gov/pubmed/21596051.

132   Institute of Medicine, *Dietary Reference Intakes*, 313, 269: "The ingestion of fat and protein has been shown to decrease the GI of foods"; "Voluntary energy intake was 29 percent higher following consumption of high GI (glycemic index) test meals."

133   Ibid., 63, "Reducing the glycemic index of a meal can result in short-term improved glucose tolerance and insulin sensitivity."

According to Dr. Sears[134] and others, a healthy division of *calories* for all meals, including breakfast, is 40 percent carbohydrates, 30 percent proteins, and 30 percent fats (more on this in the section on macro-nutrients). This is considered modestly low in carbohydrates, as in the general population, the median intake of carbohydrates is 50 percent.[135] And it is in line with one of Maimonides's guiding principles in life to generally avoid extremism—such as the Atkins extremely low car-bohydrate recommendation of 10 percent. Leaning toward low-carbo-hydrate diets without going to an extreme will protect you from high blood sugar, insulin resistance, and hyperinsulinemia.

Keep in mind that one gram of carbohydrates or protein equals four calories, whereas one gram of fat equals nine calories. You do not need to adhere to the proportionality of macronutrients with extreme precision, but you should not go below the minimal nutritional re-quirements of protein, carbohydrates, and fats. Your total caloric intake should be appropriate, and your macronutrients should be combined so that they are absorbed slowly and steadily. Macronutrient division also has a strong influence on insulin sensitivity, blood sugar stability, and weight loss or gain, which is elaborated on in chapters 10 and 14.

CONCLUSION

While it's correct not to skip breakfast, the popular recommendation to eat a full breakfast within one hour of waking is not justified when considering the physiological principles and studies in relation to insu-lin resistance and the circadian rhythm of the hormone cortisol. The hormone cortisol is at its highest daily levels shortly after waking up. Cortisol is an antagonist of insulin. It will provide you with energy via burning fat if you just allow it to work without giving yourself a shock of high blood sugar too early in the morning. If breakfast is eaten too early, the combination of cortisol and carbohydrates will spike blood sugar levels, forcing the secretion of loads of insulin. Once blood sugar

---

134   Barry Sears, *Enter the Zone* (HarperCollins, 1995), 71.
135   Institute of Medicine, *Dietary Reference Intakes*, 294–95.

levels drop, the hormones that are released to raise it back up again won't be effective because of too much insulin, leading to sugar lows, weakness, and hunger. Another problem is that a chronic simultaneous combination of raised cortisol and insulin leads to an increased fat cell number. It is better to wait to eat a full breakfast (balanced with plenty of protein and fiber and some healthy fats) until three to six hours after getting up.

Depending on one's schedule, you could manage with one or two prebreakfast snacks, eating your first meal (breakfast) during one's job's lunch break. Or, if the job's morning coffee break works out being three to four hours after the time you wake up, that might be an opportune time to schedule your daily breakfast.

Appendix to Chapter 7

Late Breakfast: The Moral Significance According to the Talmud

In the Talmudic passage that teaches the healthiest time frame within which to eat breakfast, the Talmud hints at the bond that links physical with spiritual health, and how they parallel each other. While this book is focused on physical health, spiritual health cannot be entirely ignored as it also effects physical health. As such, we have included this appendix which brings to light both the physical and spiritual aspects of this Talmudic passage.

In regard to breakfast, the Talmud[136] relates that

1. cannibals eat their breakfast upon awakening;
2. bandits eat it an hour or two after waking up;
3. "loafers" eat two to three hours after getting up;
4. normal people eat three to four hours after waking;
5. high achievers wait four to five hours; and
6. selfless, pious sages wait five to six hours.

There are many ways to understand this Talmudic passage. I extract from this two teachings that are most relevant to our present discussion.

---

136 *Talmud*, Tractate Pesachim 12b, and Tractate Shabbas 10a.

1. **Physical health**: the physiological and endocrinology-based reasons for having breakfast three to six hours after waking up have already been explained.
2. **Spiritual health, in respect to morality**: Our spiritual health affects our emotions and physical health; spirituality and physicality are two sides of one coin.

The following will elaborate on the principle hinted at in this Talmudic passage; that the key to spirituality is striving to benefit others, as opposed to striving for self-indulgence.

Some people live for the enjoyment of physical lusts, while others maintain their bodies to serve others. Viewed in the extremes are the cannibals versus the saintly people. Most people fall somewhere in-between, with varying levels of asceticism and narcissistic licentiousness.

Upon wakening, we can ask ourselves, "In which direction do I choose to live today? Self-indulgence, or being kind to others?"

For our spiritual well-being, which ultimately affects our emotions and physical health, it is best to be motivated by self-imposed goals that benefit others. This enables us to see our bodies as a tool for achieving our spiritual goals and feed it as we would feed a horse that we need to ride—in the way that will make it the strongest—as opposed to being servants to our taste buds and stomach growlings, and feeding our bodies for fleeting pleasures instead of for health.

Take note of the gradations of morality and spirituality involved in the following descriptions taken from the above passage of the Talmud:

- **Cannibals**: people who eat other people. The lowest, most selfish manner to sustain one's existence.
- **Bandits**: people with a lesser level of depravity, sustaining themselves upon others' property as opposed to others' blood.
- **Loafers**: people who don't engage in activities for the benefit of others but at least are not actively sustaining themselves in a criminal manner.

- **Normal people**: people involved in their own pleasures but also involved in benefiting others.
- **High achievers**: people who labor to better the world and help others, minimizing self-indulgence.
- **Selfless pious sages**: people completely aloof from any aspect of self-service, indulgence, or lust (I actually know of two such people, but they are very rare).

Two thousand years ago, Hillel the Sage summarized the best spiritual advice in one brief sentence, quoting the Biblical verse Leviticus 19:18:

Love your friend as yourself.

That is the force behind all of Jewish law and custom, guiding thought, speech, and action.

8

Measured Glycemic Load: Avoiding Hyperinsulinemia

Measured glycemic load is the last of the four primary elements that cures one from the metabolic syndrome. Whereas the other three elements remedy through *meal timing* and exercise, this element remedies via *meal content*—avoiding hyperinsulinemia by limiting carbohydrates both in quantity and in type and replacing carbohydrate calories with fat and protein calories.

This chapter explains the following:

- Avoiding Hyperinsulinemia
- Glycemic Index
- Glycemic Load
- Insulin Index
- Benefits of Insulin
- The Paradox of Proteins Lowering Blood Sugar yet Raising Insulin Levels
- Satiety Index

AVOIDING HYPERINSULINEMIA

Insulin is the main culprit in gaining body fat, as it directs the liver to convert excess glucose into fat and prevents the release of fat from storage for use as fuel. Most overweight people suffer from hyperinsulinemia—too much insulin. Prolonged hyperinsulinemia leads to accumulation of excess body fat, promotes diabetes, and can speed up the development of heart disease.

Concerning meal content, there are at least three factors that minimize insulin secretion:

1. **Eating a measured quantity of carbohydrates:** As previously mentioned, Dr. Sears and others recommend a macronutrient caloric division of 40 percent carbohydrates, 30 percent protein, and 30 percent fat, which is balanced and easy to follow yet significantly lower in carbohydrates than the typical 50 percent carbohydrate diet.

2. **Combining carbohydrates with fats and fiber:** Another factor in stabilizing blood sugar levels to avoid hyperinsulinemia is to slow down the absorption of carbohydrates into the blood by ingesting them together with fiber and fat, rather than having a meal or snack of just carbohydrates and having the fats and fiber at a later meal or snack.

3. **Choosing low glycemic carbohydrates:** This chapter focuses on yet another way of avoiding blood sugar spikes—choosing carbohydrates with a low glycemic index, which means they are absorbed into the blood at a slower rate than other carbs.

GLYCEMIC INDEX

The *glycemic index*, or GI, ranks foods on a scale of 0 to 100 based on how quickly they raise blood sugar levels. Foods that raise blood sugar quickly have a higher number, whereas foods that take longer to raise blood sugar levels have a lower number.

GI is categorized as either *low* (55 or less), *medium* (56–69), or *high* (70–100).

Keep in mind that the GI is imprecise. One type of apple will have a different GI than another. The GI is also affected by the way the food is prepared (the longer it is cooked, the higher the GI) and by the combination of foods it is ingested with as well as each individual person's particular response. Food processing raises the GI: for example, juice has a higher GI than whole fruit, a mashed potato has a higher GI than a whole baked potato, and regular processed whole wheat bread has a higher GI than stone-ground bread.

Additional information, GI, and glycemic load values of particular foods can be found at www.glycemicindex.com.

Proteins (meat, poultry, fish, and certain dairy products) and fats don't have a GI because they do not contain carbohydrates.

The following list of foods and their corresponding GI category is from the American Diabetes Association:[137]

Low-GI Foods (55 or less)
- One hundred percent stone-ground whole wheat and pumpernickel bread
- Oatmeal (rolled or steel cut), oat bran, and muesli
- Pasta, converted rice, barley, bulgur, and bran cereal
- Sweet potatoes, corn, yams, lima or butter beans, peas, legumes, and lentils
- Most fruits, nonstarchy vegetables, and carrots

Medium-GI Foods (56–69)
- Whole wheat, rye, and pita breads
- Quick oats
- Brown, wild, or basmati rice and couscous

High-GI Foods (70–100)
- White bread and bagels
- Corn flakes, puffed rice, bran flakes, and instant oatmeal

---

137 "Glycemic Index and Diabetes," American Diabetes Association, last modified May 14, 2004, http://www.diabetes.org/food-and-fitness/food/what-can-i-eat/understanding-carbohydrates/glycemic-index-and-diabetes.html.

- Short-grain white rice, rice pasta, and macaroni and cheese from a mix
- Russet potatoes and pumpkins
- Pretzels, rice cakes, popcorn, and saltine crackers
- Melons and pineapple

GLYCEMIC LOAD

Whereas the GI compares the speed at which various carbohydrates raise blood sugar levels, the quantity of carbohydrates has even more of an effect on raising blood sugar. The measurement of the GI multiplied by the number of grams of carbohydrates ingested divided by 100 gives us the *glycemic load*. The glycemic load of a portion of food is considered a better indicator of the overall effect of a food on blood sugar levels, because foods vary in how much carbohydrate they contain.

For example, a watermelon has a high GI of 72, but a typical one-hundred-gram serving of it only contains five grams of carbohydrate, as it is mostly water. Therefore, the glycemic load of a hundred-gram serving is only $72 \times 5 = 360 \div 100 = 3.6$ glycemic load.

Examples of how to calculate the glycemic load for different foods follow:

- **A half-cup serving of raw carrots** (about 8.6 grams of available carbohydrates and a GI of 45): $45 \times 8.6 = 387 \div 100 = \mathbf{3.9}$ glycemic load
- **Two-thirds cup of white rice** (about 36 grams of available carbohydrates and a GI of 72): $72 \times 36 = 2,592 \div 100 = \mathbf{26}$ glycemic load
- **Two-thirds cup of brown rice** (about 32 grams of available carbohydrates and a GI of 50): $50 \times 32 = 1600 \div 100 = \mathbf{16}$ glycemic load

Glycemic load is ranked as *low* (10 or less), *medium* (11–19), or *high* (20 or more).

INSULIN INDEX

The *insulin index* is a measure used to quantify the typical insulin response to various foods. The index is similar to the GI and glycemic load, but rather than relying on blood glucose levels, the insulin index is based upon blood insulin levels. This measure can be more useful than either the GI or glycemic load because certain foods (meats and other proteins) cause an insulin response despite having no carbohydrates, and some foods cause a disproportionate insulin response relative to their carbohydrate load.

BENEFITS OF INSULIN

Insulin spikes aren't always detrimental. Once a person is healed from hyperinsulinemia, if the glycogen (carbohydrate) storage in his or her muscles and liver is not full, the spike in blood sugar levels inducing a strong insulin response can at times be helpful. Insulin speeds the cellular uptake not only of sugar but also of protein and other nutrients. When a person is in a state of exhaustion after intense and extended physical activity, insulin can speed recovery and help build muscle.

THE PARADOX OF PROTEINS LOWERING
BLOOD SUGAR YET RAISING INSULIN LEVELS

For the liver to be in the mode of converting fat to sugar to be burned as energy, as opposed to being in the mode of converting sugar to fat to be stored in our fat cells, the hormonal balance needs to be such that adrenalin, cortisol, glucagon, and growth hormone outweigh the effects of insulin.

Protein stimulates the release of glucagon,[138] and carbohydrates stimulate the release of insulin. Since protein reduces the blood sugar rise from the carbohydrates,[139] one might reason that combining carbohydrates with proteins would lower the insulin response. However, protein

---

138 M. Claessens, W. H. Saris, and M. A. van Baak, "Glucagon and Insulin Responses after Ingestion of Different Amounts of Intact and Hydrolysed Proteins," *British Journal of Nutrition* (2008), http://www.ncbi.nlm.nih.gov/pubmed/18167171.

139 Frank Q. Nuttall et al., "Effect of Protein Ingestion on the Glucose and Insulin Response to a Standardized Oral Glucose Load," *Diabetes Care* (1984), http://care.diabetes-journals.org/content/7/5/465.

also induces an insulin response—certain amino acids more than others.[140] And proteins in combination with carbohydrates induce a much greater insulin response than either alone.[141] *The paradox is that adding proteins to a carbohydrate meal will lower glucose levels, while raising insulin levels.*[142]

Therefore, if the objective is to reduce the insulin response to meals, you should avoid eating large amounts of carbohydrates and proteins together in the same meal. Meals should either be primarily carbohydrates and fats or proteins and fats. If the objective is to avoid high blood sugar, combining carbohydrates with proteins will help. And if the objective is to attain the anabolic effect of increased insulin to enhance recovery and muscle building after a workout, combining carbohydrates and proteins is advantageous.

SATIETY INDEX

Another related factor that can help us choose the foods that will lead to reaching our fat-burning goals is how satisfying each particular food is per calorie. Some foods can satisfy us with fewer calories.

A study measuring the satiety levels of 240-calorie portions of thirty-eight different foods concludes that boiled potatoes are the most satisfying food per calorie; in general, the foods that weigh the most per calorie satisfy our hunger best.[143] Foods that contain large amounts of fat, sugar, and/or starch have low *fullness factors*. Foods that contain large amounts of water, dietary fiber, and/or protein (most vegetables, fruits, and lean meats, poultry, and fish) have the highest *fullness factors*.

---

140 L. J. van Loon et al., "Plasma Insulin Responses after Ingestion of Different Amino Acid or Protein Mixtures with Carbohydrate," *American Journal of Clinical Nutrition* (2000), http://ajcn.nutrition.org/content/72/1/96.long.

141 Luc J. C. van Loon et al., "Amino Acid Ingestion Strongly Enhances Insulin Secretion in Patients with Long-Term Type 2 Diabetes," *Diabetes Care* (2003), http://care.diabetes-journals.org/content/26/3/625.full.

142 Nuttall et al., "Effect of Protein Ingestion on the Glucose and Insulin Response to a Standardized Oral Glucose Load," Diabetes Care (1984), http://care.diabetesjournals.org/content/26/3/625.full.

143 S. H. Holt et al., "A Satiety Index of Common Foods," *European Journal of Clinical Nutrition* (1995), http://www.ncbi.nlm.nih.gov/pubmed/7498104.

You can find more details of their study here: http://nutritiondata.self.com/topics/fullness-factor.

The following list shows values of the fullness factor for a few common foods:

Bean sprouts	4.6	
Watermelon	4.5	
Grapefruit	4.0	
Carrots	3.8	
Oranges	3.5	
Fish, broiled	3.4	
Chicken breast, roasted	3.3	
Apples	3.3	
Sirloin steak, broiled	3.2	
Oatmeal	3.0	
Popcorn	2.9	
Baked potato	2.5	↑
Low-fat yogurt	2.5	More filling
Banana	2.5	per calorie
Macaroni and cheese	2.5	
Brown rice	2.3	Less filling
Spaghetti	2.2	per calorie
White rice	2.1	
Pizza	2.1	↓
Peanuts	2.0	
Ice cream	1.8	
White bread	1.8	
Raisins	1.6	
Snickers Bar	1.5	
Honey	1.4	
Sugar (sucrose)	1.3	
Glucose	1.3	
Potato chips	1.2	
Butter	0.5	

CONCLUSION

Although there can be exceptions to the rule, in general we want to avoid spiking blood sugar levels. Some ways of doing that are to avoid high GI foods such as white bread, Corn flakes, puffed rice, bran flakes, instant oatmeal, short-grain white rice, pretzels, rice cakes, popcorn, and crackers. Additionally many high GI foods are not very satisfying, such as sweets in particular, which leads to eating more calories, more carbohydrates, and spiking blood sugar levels. Therefore we need to be careful to minimize dependence on such foods.

9

Daily Intermittent Fasting

Intermittent fasting is an umbrella term for various diets that cycle between periods of fasting and not fasting. In respect to Maimonides's recommendations, intermittent fasting is really a side product of two of the four primary elements used to cure the metabolic syndrome—early dinner and late breakfast. Once you are acclimated to a daily routine of an extended overnight fast, you begin to reap many health benefits, as explained shortly. This chapter explains the following:

- How Many Hours of Fasting Are Ideal?
- The Importance of Adapting Gradually
- The Benefits of Daily Intermittent Fasting
- Detoxification via Prolonged Fasting
- Fasting is Not Starvation or Malnutrition
- Intermittent Fasting Compared to Continuous Fasting

HOW MANY HOURS OF FASTING ARE IDEAL?

Maimonides advises not to ingest anything but water later than three to four hours before bedtime. The Talmud advises (and Maimonides agrees) not to have breakfast before three hours after arising from bed. Since Maimonides recommends sleeping seven to eight hours, the daily recommended intermittent fast lasts at least thirteen hours. Considering that it is healthy to have breakfast as late as six hours after waking, the daily interval for abstinence could be as much as eighteen hours. Therefore the healthy and moderate recommended daily fast is between fourteen and sixteen hours, leaving a window of eight to ten hours for ingesting and absorbing all the nutrients you need to maintain health.

Limiting the time for food indulgences to a mere ten hours may appear as deprivation and unappealing, but the health of the body must be maintained to maximize its abilities to function.

THE IMPORTANCE OF ADAPTING GRADUALLY

People who are accustomed to eating late at night and/or early in the morning should realize that making drastic sudden changes in their lifestyle is likely to be harmful. Rather, you should gradually acclimate yourself to the healthier lifestyle of resting your digestive system fourteen to sixteen consecutive hours a day.

THE BENEFITS OF DAILY INTERMITTENT FASTING

Daily intermittent fasting has many health benefits, including the following:

1. **Enables the burning of fat.** Studies demonstrate that intermittent fasting decreases body fat, LDL cholesterol, and triacylglycerol concentrations.[144] A great advantage of intermittent fasting is that it enables the body to maximize its fat-burning abilities fifteen hours per day. When done correctly, according to Maimonides's prescriptions, your daily fast should begin three to four hours before bedtime and end three to six hours after awakening. This schedule takes advantage of the body's natural hormonal daily cycle of fat-burning hormones kicking in at night, when people normally sleep and lack energy originating from food in the intestinal tract. Accustoming yourself

---

144 Krista A. Varady et al., "Short-Term Modified Alternate-Day Fasting: A Novel Dietary Strategy for Weight Loss and Cardioprotection in Obese Adults," *American Journal of Clinical Nutrition* (2009), http://ajcn.nutrition.org/content/90/5/1138.

to daily fasts and building them up to fifteen to sixteen hours per day trains you to stretch out the daily fat-burning window. When glycogen (sugar) stores are low, the body speeds up fat burning in attempt to prevent using up all the sugar reserves.[145] The longer the fast, the lower the glycogen stores, and the faster the body burns fat. Yet maintaining the eight-hour window for daily food consumption avoids the harm of going too long without food, as prolonged fasting weakens the body, slows metabolism, and consumes muscle for sustenance.

2. **Lowers blood pressure**. Studies demonstrate that intermittent fasting lowers blood pressure.[146]

3. **Avoids bad digestion**. Sleep inhibits digestion, as digestion is dependent on blood flow and body movement, which are greatly reduced during sleep. Food that is eaten too late does not get digested properly and can cause toxic reactions and gases. And digestive acids linger for hours in the same spot. Sleeping on an empty stomach avoids these harmful effects. Therefore, beginning one's daily intermittent fast a few hours before bedtime has the advantage of protecting the digestive system.

4. **Enables deep sleep and secretion of HGH**. Digestion inhibits sleep. When the digestive tract and the liver are required to work to process food, they demand higher blood concentration, pressure, and flow, thereby disrupting the rest of the cardiovascular system. Failing to have deep sleep inhibits the secretion of HGH—human growth hormone. In contrast, if you sleep on an empty stomach, the digestive tract, liver, and cardiovascular systems can rest, and the body can benefit from deeper sleep and maximal secretion of HGH, which contributes to revitalizing our bodies at night. HGH is lypolytic (stimulates the burning of

---

145 Katarina T. Borer, "Advanced Exercise Endocrinology," *Human Kinetics* (2013): 106.
146 Varady et al., "Short-Term Modified Alternate-Day Fasting: A Novel Dietary Strategy for Weight Loss and Cardioprotection in Obese Adults," *American Journal of Clinical Nutrition* (2009), http://ajcn.nutrition.org/content/90/5/1138.

visceral fats for energy) and also triggers the release of insulin-like growth factor (IGF-1), which is a primary mediator of muscle repair and growth. Artificial HGH treatment has negligible benefits aside from fat loss; however, the use of a synthetic form of growth-hormone-releasing hormone (GHRH), which stimulates the body's *natural* release of HGH, yields significant benefits. It restores normal HGH pulsation and amplitude, increasing IGF-1 to upper physiologic ranges; selectively reduces abdominal visceral adipose tissue, cIMT, CRP, and triglycerides; and improves cognitive function in older persons.[147] (Increased values of cIMT carotid intima-media thickness [the thickness of the inner two layers of the carotid artery—the intima and media], and high-sensitivity C-reactive protein CRP [a marker of inflammation that predicts incident myocardial infarction, stroke, peripheral arterial disease, and sudden cardiac death among healthy individuals with no history of cardiovascular disease, and recurrent events and death in patients with acute or stable coronary syndromes]—are predictors of acute coronary events).

5. **Avoids inhibition of HGH by avoiding insulin secretion at night.** When you eat late-night meals that include carbohydrates, it causes your body to secrete insulin. Insulin inhibits the secretion of HGH and inhibits the beneficial effects of whatever HGH is secreted. By going to sleep on an empty stomach, we enable our bodies to secrete and fully utilize the incredible revitalizing benefits of HGH.

6. **Avoids the ills of hyperinsulinemia.** In a study by the Salk Institute for Biological Studies,[148] two groups of mice were compared; one group was allowed to eat twenty-four hours a day, and the other group ate the same type of food, with the

---

147 Fred R. Sattler, "Growth Hormone in the Aging Male," *Clinical Endocrinological Metabolism* (August 2013), http://www.ncbi.nlm.nih.gov/pmc/articles/PMC3940699/.

148 Megumi Hatori et al., "Time-Restricted Feeding without Reducing Caloric Intake Prevents Metabolic Diseases in Mice Fed a High-Fat Diet," *Cell Metabolism* 15, no. 6 (June 6, 2012): 848–60, http://www.cell.com/cell-metabolism/abstract/S1550-4131(12)00189-1.

same caloric intake, but the group's eating was restricted to an eight-hour period with sixteen hours per day of involuntary fasting. The intermittent-fasting mice showed improved insulin sensitivity (protection from hyperinsulinemia) and were protected from obesity.

The above study on mice doesn't prove that intermittent fasting would help hyperinsulinemia in humans; however, a small study on eight healthy men who fasted for twenty-hour intervals every other day for two weeks, while eating enough to maintain their body weight, demonstrates that the intermittent fasting improved insulin sensitivity in humans.[149]

A similar study of eight men and eight women fasting on alternate days for three weeks also demonstrates improved insulin sensitivity and weight loss; however, the researchers concluded that the participants' perpetual hunger on the fasting days made it too difficult to adapt to as a lifestyle.[150] Unlike the difficult twenty-four-hour fasts of this study, gradually adjusting to the Maimonides method of daily, sixteen-hour overnight fasts is not too difficult to adapt to as a lifestyle. Surprisingly, the reduced appetite that becomes habituated with daily intermittent fasting is often more comfortable than dealing with uncontrollable constant urges.

Another six-month study of 107 obese women compares the effects of intermittent energy restriction to continuous energy restriction and concludes that "intermittent energy restriction is more effective in reducing hyperinsulinemia."[151]

---

149 Nils Halberg et al., "Effect of Intermittent Fasting and Refeeding on Insulin Action in Healthy Men," *Journal of Applied Physiology* 99, no. 6 (December 2005), 2128–36, http://jap.physiology.org/content/99/6/2128

150 L. K. Heilbronn et al., "Alternate-Day Fasting in Nonobese Subjects: Effects on Body Weight, Body Composition, and Energy Metabolism," *American Journal of Clinical Nutrition* (2005), http://ajcn.nutrition.org/content/81/1/69.full.pdf+html.

151 Michelle N. Harvie et al., "The Effects of Intermittent or Continuous Energy Restriction on Weight Loss and Metabolic Disease Risk Markers: A Randomised Trial in Young Overweight Women," *International Journal of Obesity* (May 2011), http://www.ncbi.nlm.nih.gov/pmc/articles/PMC3017674/.

Intermittent fasting of more than twelve hours is guaranteed to deplete glycogen reserves in the liver (also in the muscle to a lesser extent) such that those tissues will be prepared to respond quickly to insulin, absorbing sugar from the blood. As catabolic hormones are at their daily peak shortly after awakening, those hormones oppose insulin and cause insulin resistance. Waiting for breakfast until those hormones subside will enable the body to respond well to insulin when breaking the fast with one's first meal of the day. By avoiding the pitfalls of hyperinsulinemia, you avoid the onset of hunger pangs, overeating, and the conversion of carbohydrates to excess body fat.

7. **Enables control of total daily caloric intake.** For people suffering from obesity, having more hours in the day to eat means more hours to struggle with temptations and maintain control. Habituating oneself to limit the window of eating makes it easier to control daily caloric intake.

8. **Enables detoxification.** While digesting food, the body accumulates toxins. When the digestive tract rests, the body removes them. However, the detoxifying process requires a lot of time, because on the cellular level, the anabolic processes of utilizing the digested nutrients goes on for hours after the initial digestion of the food. The body can manage some detoxifying processes virtually all the time, but the effectiveness increases as the length of the fast increases. The main benefits of detoxification occur in the last three to four hours of the daily overnight fast of fourteen to sixteen hours.

9. **Intensifies autophagy.** Intermittent fasting also intensifies the body's natural process of autophagy[152, 153]—the controlled

---

152   M. Alirezaei et al., "Short-Term Fasting Induces Profound Neuronal Autophagy," *Autophagy (August 2010), http://www.ncbi.nlm.nih.gov/pubmed/20534972.*

153   I. Kim and J. J. Lemasters, "Mitochondrial Degradation by Autophagy (Mitophagy) in GFP-LC3 Transgenic Hepatocytes during Nutrient Deprivation," *American Journal of Physiology, Cell Physiology* (February 2011), http://www.ncbi.nlm.nih.gov/pubmed/21106691.

destruction of damaged organelles within a cell, which has been shown to have anti-aging effects[154]—and is required to maintain muscle mass.[155]

10. **Prolongs life.** With all these health benefits, intermittent fasting should lead to a healthier and longer life. Studies on mice clearly demonstrate that intermittent fasting lengthens life.[156]

DETOXIFICATION VIA PROLONGED FASTING

The Maimonides method of diet incorporates daily intermittent fasting. Longer term fasting of several days or weeks has been used as a method of rehabilitation at times through its power of detoxification. By examining the benefits of extended fasting, we can better understand the similar benefits of daily intermittent fasting. Here's what people are saying about extended fasting:

> A little starvation can really do more for the average sick man than can the best of medicines and the best doctors. I do not mean a restricted diet: I mean total abstinence from food.
>
> —Mark Twain

In *Fasting and Eating for Health*, Dr. Joel Fuhrman gives examples of the healing power of fasting by observing the behavior of sick or injured animals. Instinctively, they only sip water while resting until their health is restored. He explains the healing process of fasting as a drop

---

154 E. Bergamini et al., "The Role of Autophagy in Aging: Its Essential Part in the Anti-Aging Mechanism of Caloric Restriction," *Annals of the New York Academy of Sciences* (2007), http://www.ncbi.nlm.nih.gov/pubmed/17934054.

155 E. Masiero et al., "Autophagy Is Required to Maintain Muscle Mass," *Cell Metabolism* (2009), http://www.ncbi.nlm.nih.gov/pubmed/19945408.

156 J. A. Carlson and F. Hoelzel, "Apparent Prolongation of the Life Span of Rats by Intermittent Fasting," *Journal of Nutrition* (1946), *http://www.ncbi.nlm.nih.gov/pubmed/21021020.*

in blood pressure, with less retention of metabolic wastes, a softening of the blood vessels via ridding themselves of hard sclerotic plaque, and a purification of body tissue. The fast forces the body to search within itself for sources of energy, and through the wisdom of nature, it chooses to consume needless tissue; in this process of "self-digestion," the body consumes and destroys fat, tumors, blood vessel plaque, and diseased tissue.

According to Dr. Fuhrman, medical studies show that fasting is therapeutic for the liver, psychological disorders, and brain function and alleviates neuroses, anxiety, and depression. He writes that according to many scientists, aging is largely due to toxins accumulating inside of cells, causing internal cell damage and reducing cellular function. Fasting is, of course, detoxifying, and as such it helps to maintain our youth and vitality.

FASTING IS NOT STARVATION OR MALNUTRITION

Fasting should not be confused with starvation or chronic malnutrition. During fasting, the body cleanses itself of everything except vital tissue. During starvation, the body is forced to use vital tissue to survive. Malnutrition results from eating a diet in which certain nutrients are lacking, in excess, or in the wrong proportions. Chronic malnutrition usually happens when eating the wrong foods over extended time. When a *healthy* person fasts, the body has reserves of all the minerals and nutrients that it needs to easily survive one or two months before those reserves are depleted.

In extended fasts, much muscle is lost, since the body consumes muscle as a source of fuel. During the first three days of total fasting, muscle consumption is very intense. After that, the body adapts to the fast by surviving on ketones (a by-product of the breakdown of stored fats) instead of glucose and consumes much smaller amounts of muscle.

In summary, the main advantage of fasting is cleansing the body. The main disadvantage of extended fasting is the loss of muscle.

INTERMITTENT FASTING COMPARED TO CONTINUOUS FASTING

One purpose of intermittent fasting is to gain the benefit—cleansing—while avoiding the muscle loss that is associated with continuous fasting.

With daily fifteen-hour fasts paralleled by nine-hour daily windows for eating, it is possible to supply the body with all the needed nutrition, even during intensive training programs that require the greatest-possible absorption of nutrients to develop strength and muscle. In fact, intermittent fasting has been shown to improve muscle development.[157]

Fasting intermittently also has numerous benefits that are not obtained with continuous fasts, such as promoting insulin sensitivity, improving sleep, elevating HGH levels, and improving the health of the digestive tract.

CONCLUSION

By expanding our overnight fast—beginning it earlier and ending it later—we attain daily intermittent fasting, yielding these benefits:

1. Burning off fat
2. Avoiding the harmful effects of bad digestion
3. Increasing deep sleep and secretion of HGH
4. Avoiding inhibition of HGH by avoiding insulin secretion at night
5. Promoting insulin sensitivity
6. Assisting in limiting calorie intake
7. Cleansing the body of toxins

Yet, when properly scheduled, the nine-hour window of eating provides sufficient time to digest and absorb all the necessary nutrients for sustenance and growth, thus avoiding the consumption of muscle tissue that occurs in extended fasts.

---

157 E Masiero et al., "Autophagy Is Required to Maintain Muscle Mass," *Cell Metabolism* (2009), http://www.ncbi.nlm.nih.gov/pubmed/19945408.

Part III

Macronutrients

What the Body Uses Them for, Recommended Sources, How Much We Need, and Planning a Healthy and Balanced Diet

10

RDA of Macronutrients (Carbohydrates, Proteins, and Fats)

In chapter 4, I listed four primary elements for alleviating the metabolic syndrome: early dinner, exercise, late breakfast, and measured glycemic load. For most people, a measured glycemic load includes a reduction in carbohydrates and limiting high-GI carbohydrates. A reduction in carbohydrates needs to be balanced by an increase in fats and/or proteins.

This chapter explains the basics about the three different macronutrients, the minimum requirements, and the controversy surrounding the RDA—recommended daily allowances.

MACRONUTRIENTS: MINIMUM REQUIREMENTS

Macronutrients are nutrients that are required in larger amounts compared to micronutrients. Macronutrients provide calories, or energy, and consist of carbohydrates, proteins, and fats. Carbohydrates and proteins supply four calories per gram, and fat supplies nine calories per gram.

Carbohydrates

Carbohydrates are either simple sugars or complex chains of sugars that can be hydrolyzed (broken down) into simple sugars. Even though the body depends on carbohydrates to function (the brain and nervous system are especially dependent upon glucose—blood sugar), carbohydrates are not "essential" (needed in your diet) because the body can alternatively convert proteins and fats into glucose. However, deficiencies in dietary fiber, a type of carbohydrate, are linked to a higher risk of numerous types of cancers, heart disease, and diabetes.[158] As such, the RDA (recommended daily allowance) of fiber is fourteen grams per one thousand calories of intake—roughly thirty-two grams for the average adult. Considering that various types of fibers provide between zero and 2.5 calories per gram, thirty-two grams of fiber would provide approximately thirty-two calories. Additionally, without a minimal consumption of carbohydrates, there would most likely be deficiencies in micronutrients such as vitamin C and certain B vitamins.

Fats

In general, fats are not essential, with the exception of omega-3 and omega-6. One gram per day (nine calories) of omega-3 fish oils (EPA, DHA) is sufficient, but more is usually better. Although omega-6 is essential, we need to minimize our intake since the typical diet includes too much, actually making it harmful. Even though the body can manufacture most of the fats it needs, nevertheless, dietary fats are crucial in the absorption of numerous important micronutrients: zinc, vitamins A and K-2, and certain B vitamins. Below ten grams per day (ninety calories) of fat intake is likely to lead to deficiencies in these micronutrients, whereas more than ten grams does not provide further benefit.[159]

Protein

Proteins are essential. Aside from the fact that nine or ten amino acids cannot be produced (either sufficiently or at all) by the body from other amino acids, digesting less than the RDA of 0.80 grams of quality protein per kilogram of body weight (roughly fifty grams daily for the average

---

158 Institute of Medicine, *Dietary Reference Intakes*, 366–96.
159 Ibid., 785–8.

adult—two hundred calories) can lead to deficiencies. Additionally, since certain essential nutrients such as long-chain omega-3 fatty acids, iron, zinc, and vitamin B-12 are more abundant in animal-derived foods, a deficiency in protein would most likely lead to deficiencies in other essential nutrients.

Macronutrient Division

The average adult needs in the vicinity of 1800 to 2800 calories a day for energy balance, and the minimal requirements of the respective macronutrients total only 322 calories a day (10 g [90 cal] of fats, including omega-3; 50 g [200 cal] of protein; and 32 g [32 cal] of fiber equals 322 cal). Therefore, there is plenty of leeway in how individuals can choose to distribute their macronutrient intake.

MACRONUTRIENTS: ACCEPTABLE RANGE ACCORDING TO THE IOM

According to the Institute of Medicine (IOM),[160] the acceptable macronutrient distribution range for adults is as follows:

- **Carbohydrates**: 45–65 percent
- **Proteins**: 10–35 percent
- **Fats**: 20–35 percent

The IOM is a branch of the National Academy of Sciences authorized by Congress in 1863 to advise the government on scientific matters. Its 1,331-page book on diet recommendations, *Dietary Reference Intakes*, or the DRI, was written and edited by a team of over fifty university professors and doctors. Congress has authorized the IOM to determine the standard dietary guidelines, and since many places prohibit giving diet recommendations without being licensed, the IOM guidelines have effectively become law.

---

160 Institute of Medicine, *Dietary Reference Intakes*, (National Academies Press, (2005), 1325.

CONTRADICTORY STATEMENTS OF THE IOM CONCERNING ACCEPTABLE CARBOHYDRATE INTAKE

There appears to me to be numerous contradictions in the IOM's 1,331 pages on macronutrient diet recommendations. With so many contributing authors, this can be expected; however, what strikes me as the most problematic are the contradictions regarding a high-carbohydrate diet and setting of the acceptable range of carbohydrates between 45 and 65 percent of total caloric intake.

Take, for example, this apparent contradiction: in regard to carbohydrate consumption and diabetes, the IOM writes, "There is little evidence that total dietary carbohydrate intake is associated with type 2 diabetes."[161]

This seems to contradict some other statements of the IOM: "The ingestion of fat and protein has been shown to decrease the GI of foods"[162] and "Reducing the glycemic index of a meal can result in short-term improved glucose tolerance and insulin sensitivity."[163] In other words, replacing carbohydrates with proteins and fats will reduce the glycemic index of a meal and improve insulin sensitivity, thereby stabilizing blood sugar levels.

Furthermore, the IOM writes that high GI (Glycemic Index) meals increase appetite (high GI foods are carbohydrates—fats and proteins don't have any GI): "Voluntary energy intake was 29 percent higher following consumption of high GI (Glycemic Index) test meals."[164]

Obviously eating more leads to obesity, and the IOM explains that obesity worsens insulin resistance, thereby leading to diabetes: "Obesity is related to decreased insulin sensitivity."[165]

---

161 Ibid., 63.
162 Institute of Medicine, *Dietary Reference Intakes*, 269.
163 Ibid, 63.
164 Ibid, 313.
165 Ibid, 303.

Seeing that the IOM acknowledges in the DRI that obesity is related to decreased insulin sensitivity, it should be obvious that very low-carbohydrate diets can be quite beneficial for obese diabetics, as there are so many studies demonstrating that very low-carbohydrate diets are the most effective for short-term (up to six months) weight loss, and in the long term, they are most effective for insulin sensitivity. These facts can no longer be disputed (see chapter 14 for details of some of these studies).

Furthermore, according to the IOM,[166] controlled studies have demonstrated that *high*-GI diets result in higher LDL (bad) cholesterol levels and lower HDL (good) cholesterol levels, and the IOM writes: "High carbohydrate (low fat) intakes tend to increase plasma triacylglycerol and decrease plasma HDL,"[167] all of which increase the risk factor for heart disease.

In other words, high GI worsens insulin sensitivity; thereby

1. increasing the risk of diabetes or worsening the existing diabetes,
2. leading to obesity,
3. leading to higher LDL cholesterol levels, and
4. increasing the risk of heart disease.

In respect to the carbohydrate sugar, the IOM does recognize that increased added sugars lead to obesity and type 2 diabetes: "Increased added sugars intakes have been shown to result in increased energy intakes...For each additional serving of drinks sweetened with sugars consumed, the odds of becoming obese increased by 60 percent!"[168]

The IOM further states, "Obesity is a primary risk factor for insulin resistance and development of type 2 diabetes."[169]

---

166 Ibid, 303.
167 Ibid., 59.
168 Ibid, 312.
169 Ibid, 62.

Yet the IOM writes[170] that up to 25 percent of energy consumed can come from added sugars and up to 65 percent from carbohydrates, "as there is little evidence that total dietary carbohydrate intake is associated with type 2 diabetes."[171]

This statement not only contradicts many other statements of the IOM, but it defies logic; diabetes is a disease of high blood sugar, and proteins and fats don't raise blood sugar—carbohydrates do. People with diabetes or prediabetes have to be careful not only about minimizing high-GI carbohydrates but also about limiting all carbohydrates other than fiber.

STUDIES REFUTE THE IOM'S CLAIM

The IOM's claim that "there is little evidence that total dietary carbohydrate intake is associated with type 2 diabetes"[172] is not correct. In truth there is much evidence that total dietary carbohydrate intake is associated with type 2 diabetes. In one study[173] comparing a diet of 55 percent carbohydrates to a diet of 20 percent carbohydrates, the low-carbohydrate diet ingested for five weeks dramatically reduced the circulating glucose concentration in people with untreated type 2 diabetes. Several other studies demonstrate that very low-carbohydrate diets are beneficial in respect to improving insulin sensitivity.[174, 175] Other studies demonstrate that a low-carbohydrate diet is not only effective for improving glycemia but also

---

170   Ibid, 770.

171   Ibid, 63.

172   Ibid, 63.

173   M. C. Gannon and F. Q. Nuttall, "Effect of a High-Protein, Low-Carbohydrate Diet on Blood Glucose Control in People with Type 2 Diabetes," *Diabetes* (2004).

174   Frederick F. Samaha et al., "A Low-Carbohydrate as Compared with a Low-Fat Diet in Severe Obesity," *New England Journal of Medicine* (2003), http://www.nejm.org/doi/full/10.1056/NEJMoa022637.

175   J. S. Volek et al., "Carbohydrate Restriction Has a More Favorable Impact on the Metabolic Syndrome than a Low Fat Diet," *Lipids* (2009), http://link.springer.com/article/10.1007/s11745-008-3274-2/fulltext.html.

successfully reduces the need for medications in patients with type 2 diabetes.[176, 177, 178]

An additional study compared thirty-nine overweight young adults reducing weight by 10 percent via a restricted calorie intake, either by a low-glycemic or low-fat diet. It concluded that in the low-glycemic diet, participants were less hungry and had improved insulin sensitivity, triglyceride levels, and blood pressure, leading to the conclusion that "reduction in glycemic load may aid in the prevention or treatment of obesity, cardiovascular disease, and diabetes mellitus."[179]

HOW RELEVANT IS THE RECOMMENDED ACCEPTABLE RANGE OF CARBOHYDRATE INTAKE FOR THE PUBLIC AT LARGE?

In an attempt to justify the IOM's setting the acceptable range of carbohydrates to a high level of between 45 and 65 percent of total caloric intake, a licensed dietitian pointed out to me that the IOM explicitly writes that the RDAs are what they recommend for *healthy* individuals.[180] In other words, whereas 45 percent carbohydrates may be high for diabetics, prediabetics, obese persons, and people with cardiovascular disease, for healthy people, 45 to 65 percent is acceptable.

However, although only 9.3 percent of the total adult population has diabetes, an additional *third* of the entire adult population suffers from prediabetes (not including the 9.3 percent with full-fledged diabetes).

176   R. L. Saslow et al., "A Randomized Pilot Trial of a Moderate Carbohydrate Diet Compared with a Very Low Carbohydrate Diet in Overweight or Obese Individuals with Type 2 Diabetes Mellitus or Prediabetes," *PLoS One* 9(2014): e91027.
177   W. S. Yancy Jr. et al., "A Low-Carbohydrate, Ketogenic Diet to Treat Type 2 Diabetes," *Nutrition and Metabolism* (2005), http://www.nutritionandmetabolism.com/content/2/1/34.
178   Eric C. Westman et al., "The Effect of a Low-Carbohydrate, Ketogenic Diet versus a Low-Glycemic Index Diet on Glycemic Control in Type 2 Diabetes Mellitus," *Nutrition and Metabolism* (2008), http://www.ncbi.nlm.nih.gov/pmc/articles/PMC2633336/.
179   A. M. Pereira et al., "Effects of a Low-Glycemic Load Diet on Resting Energy Expenditure and Heart Disease Risk Factors during Weight Loss," *Journal of the American Medical Association* (2004), http://www.ncbi.nlm.nih.gov/pubmed/15562127.
180   Institute of Medicine, *Dietary Reference Intakes*, 22.

Sixteen percent of adults ages forty-five to sixty-four have diabetes, and over one-fourth of the population over sixty-five suffers from diabetes. Diabetes is the seventh-leading cause of death in the United States, and the epidemic is only getting worse each year.

According to the US Department of Health, more than two in three adults are overweight or obese, with more than one in three obese (BMI 30+).

According to the American Heart Association, 40 percent of middle-aged adults (between forty and sixty years old) suffer from cardiovascular disease.

In other words, the RDA of 45 to 65 percent for carbohydrates does *not* apply to the general population at large, because most adults are either prediabetics or diabetics, overweight or obese, suffer from cardiovascular disease, or a combination of the above. Rather, the RDA applies only to the healthy minority of the population.

THE STUMBLING BLOCK OF THE IOM RECOMMENDATION TO INCREASE CARBOHYDRATES

In the United States, the median intake of carbohydrates is 50 percent of total caloric intake.[181] By setting the acceptable range of carbohydrates between 45 to 65 percent, the IOM gives the impression that you could or should have more.

People assume that the recommendations of the IOM are for the public at large, when in fact they are intended only for healthy people to the exclusion of the vast majority of the population. Therefore the IOM has created a stumbling block, leading many people to worsen their prediabetes or diabetes, obesity, and heart conditions by relying on the IOM's recommendations.

In light of all the above, I hereby add my voice in protest of the IOM's setting the acceptable intake of carbohydrates at 45 to 65 percent.

---

181   Ibid, 294–95.

THE IOM FAILS TO ADDRESS THE EFFECTS OF SUBSTITUTING CARBOHYDRATES WITH PROTEINS IN REGARD TO OBESITY AND DIABETES

Almost all the discussion in the DRI concerning comparisons of high-carbohydrate to low-carbohydrate diets is in reference to substituting carbohydrates with fats; in other words, comparing high-carbohydrate, low-fat diets to low-carbohydrate, high-fat diets. In the entire 1,331 pages, I only found one small paragraph[182] that addresses the issue of substituting carbohydrates with proteins. In this paragraph, the institute writes that substituting protein for carbohydrates lowers blood pressure, LDL, and triacylglycerol concentrations. However, it fails to address the effects of substituting protein for carbohydrates in regard to obesity and diabetes. One four-month study[183] that the DRI neglects to mention (concerning two groups, both with a five-hundred-calorie-a-day deficit) shows that not only does the higher-protein diet reduce weight significantly more than the moderate-protein diet, but the weight loss comes more from body fat than it does in the moderate protein diet. The insulin response was also greatly improved in the high protein diet. Rather, the DRI states: "Studies on the influence of high carbohydrate diets on biomarker precursors for type 2 diabetes are lacking."[184]

MOST PEOPLE WOULD BENEFIT BY LOWERING CARBOHYDRATES AND INCREASING PROTEIN

It is true that the body can convert fats and proteins into sugar, but it is a slow process, much slower than converting carbohydrates into glucose

---

182   Ibid, 60.
183   Denise A. Walker-Lasker, Ellen M. Evans, and Donald K. Layman, "Moderate Carbohydrate, Moderate Protein Weight Loss Diet Reduces Cardiovascular Disease Risk Compared to High Carbohydrate, Low Protein Diet in Obese Adults: A Randomized Clinical Trial," *Nutrition and Metabolism* (2008). http://www.nutritionandmetabolism.com/content/5/1/30.
184   Institute of Medicine, *Dietary Reference Intakes*, 785.

and even much slower than converting low-GI carbohydrates into glucose. Therefore, for the two out of three overweight adults and nearly half the adult population with high blood sugar (9.3% have diabetes plus 32% with prediabetes), it is preferable to avoid high blood sugar by avoiding high-GI foods and high carbohydrate intake. Additionally, this sector of the population should take further steps to improve insulin sensitivity, such as exercising regularly, avoiding late night meals, and delaying breakfast.

The biggest health problem today is the metabolic syndrome—obesity, diabetes, and heart disease—and the overconsumption of carbohydrates exacerbates these problems. No wonder that the high-carbohydrate allowance of the Institute of Medicine is contested by numerous doctors: Dr. Atkins recommends perhaps the lowest amount, limiting carbohydrates to less than 10 percent of caloric intake. Dr. Barry Sears, creator of the Zone diet, says the ideal macronutrient distribution is 40 percent carbohydrates, 30 percent protein, and 30 percent fat. Dr. Loren Cordain, founder of the Paleo diet, sets the upper limit for carbohydrates at 40 percent.

A high-carbohydrate diet can be advantageous for professional athletes and for people who do hours of aerobics every day, but for others there is absolutely no necessity to consume more than 40 percent carbohydrates. Even the IOM recognizes this: "The lower limit of dietary carbohydrate compatible with life apparently is zero."[185] High-carbohydrate diets usually lead to high blood sugar levels, which cause the body to produce more cholesterol, contributing to obesity, diabetes, and cardiovascular disease.

Interestingly, the Institute of Medicine writes that several case-control studies have linked sugar-rich diets with a higher risk of colon cancer, while it associates high vegetable and fruit diets that are low on refined sugars with a lower risk of colon cancer.[186]

---

185 Institute of Medicine, *Dietary Reference Intakes*, 275.
186 Ibid., 55.

In chapter 14, I examine numerous studies that unanimously conclude that for short-term diets (six months or less), the lower the percentage of carbohydrates, the more successful the weight loss.

CONCLUSION

The median intake of carbohydrates is 50 percent of macronutrients among the general population; however, most people would be healthier by balancing their macronutrient consumption with fewer carbohydrates and more protein.

Protein

Chapter 4 explained that the fourth primary element for alleviating the metabolic syndrome is measured glycemic load. In chapter 10 I elaborated on the importance of following a diet of reduced carbohydrates. A reduction in carbohydrates needs to be balanced by an increase in fats and/or proteins. This chapter explains the following:

- The Importance of Protein
- The Minimal Amount of Protein Needed Each Day
- How Much Protein Is Too Much
- The Effects of Combining Protein with Other Foods
- When to Eat Protein and When Not to Eat Protein
- Storage of Protein in the Body
- The Importance of Eating Complete Proteins
- What Foods Constitute a Source of Complete Protein
- What Foods Are Rich in Protein
- How Much Protein Is Ideal for a Balanced Diet

THE IMPORTANCE OF PROTEIN

Except for water, proteins are the most abundant type of molecule in the body. About three-quarters of body solids are proteins—molecules involved in virtually all cell functions.

What follows are the various types of proteins and their functions:

- **Nucleoproteins (DNA and RNA)**: The *DNA* in the nuclei of our cells is responsible for storing the genetic code. *Messenger RNAs* copy the information from the DNA and bring it to the protein-synthesis section of the cell (the ribosomes). *Ribosomal RNAs* constitute about 60 percent of the ribosome structure. *Transfer RNAs* do the work of building proteins inside the ribosomes by transferring amino acids one by one to the protein chains under construction there.
- **Structural proteins**: These proteins include keratin, collagen, and elastin. Skin, hair, and nails are made primarily of *keratins*. Bones are primarily made of *collagens*. Connective tissues such as tendons and ligaments are made primarily of *elastin*.
- **Contractile proteins**: The proteins actin and myosin are responsible for muscle contraction and movement.
- **Enzymes**: These are proteins that facilitate biochemical reactions. Lactase breaks down the sugar lactose found in milk, and pepsin breaks down proteins in food.
- **Hormonal proteins**: These are messenger proteins that help to coordinate certain bodily activities.
- **Transport proteins**: These carrier proteins move molecules from one place to another around the body. Examples include hemoglobin and cytochromes. Hemoglobin transports oxygen through the blood. Cytochromes operate in the electron transport chain as electron carrier proteins.
- **Antibodies**: These specialized proteins defend against bacteria, viruses, and other foreign intruders.
- **Fuel**: Proteins can be converted to sugar to be used for fuel or stored as fat. Branched-chain amino acids can be used as fuel by muscles without being converted to sugar. Proteins contain four calories per gram, just like carbohydrates but unlike lipids, which contain nine calories per gram.

- **Precursors of nonprotein products**: These are necessary for physiological viability, such as creatine (muscle function), bile acids, thyroid hormones, and so forth.

In addition to their numerous functions, proteins also vary in structure. Proteins are constructed from a set of twenty amino acids. The body can produce certain amino acids from others; however, there are nine amino acids that are "essential"—meaning they must be attained through diet for the body to construct the proteins it needs to function and maintain itself.

Animal sources of protein include meats, dairy products, fish, and eggs. Vegetarian sources of proteins include grains, legumes, nuts, and seeds.

WHAT IS THE MINIMAL AMOUNT OF PROTEIN THAT YOU NEED TO EAT EACH DAY?

The IOM's RDA (recommended daily allowance) is 0.8 grams of protein per kilogram of body weight, or 0.36 grams per pound of body weight. The measurement is based on one's body weight, not including the excess fat, as protein is not needed to maintain excess fat. For example, a 205-pound man who is fifty pounds overweight would measure his protein requirement according to what his weight should be: 155 pounds (155 × 0.36 = 56 grams recommended daily protein). This calculation amounts to fifty-six grams of protein daily for the average sedentary adult man and forty-six grams of protein daily for the average sedentary adult woman. According to *The Textbook of Medical Physiology*, at least sixty to sixty-five grams of protein are recommended for the average adult.[187] Growing children need more protein pound for pound than adults. Likewise, women during pregnancy or when breastfeeding have higher protein requirements. The more active you are, the more protein you need. Building muscle requires lots of protein to enhance

---

187 Guyton and Hall, *Textbook of Medical Physiology* (Saunders, 2011), 835.

muscle-protein synthesis and to make up for the loss of amino acid oxidation during exercise; therefore, body builders and weight lifters are at the top of the spectrum, needing as much as two grams of protein per kilogram of body weight. Even endurance training, which does not involve muscle building, nevertheless involves an increase in the burning of BCAAs (branched chain amino acids) in the muscles, requiring an estimated 0.94 g/kg/d.[188] Those on calorie-restricted diets need to keep in mind that the previously stated RDA estimate is in respect to a caloric homeostatic diet. However, when calories are restricted, the body burns proteins to meet energy needs; therefore, a quantity of protein higher than the RDA is needed to avoid protein deficiencies. Protein deficiency has been shown to have harmful effects on the brain and adverse effects on the immune system, gut permeability, and kidney function.[189]

If one does not consume adequate protein, his or her muscle will waste away, since more vital cellular processes (e.g. respiration enzymes, blood cells) recycle muscle protein for their own requirements.

HOW MUCH PROTEIN IS TOO MUCH?

For people with healthy kidneys, the main limitation on protein consumption depends on their caloric limitation. If a person eats more protein than his or her body needs for protein synthesis and energy, the body turns some of it into lipids and stores it as body fat, while some protein the body disposes of. Therefore, the maximum amount of protein depends on one's daily caloric consumption and how many of the calories are from carbohydrates and dietary fats. For example, on a two-thousand-homeostatic-calorie diet, if five hundred calories consumed are from carbohydrates and five hundred are from lipids, one can eat one thousand calories (250 grams) of proteins without gaining weight. If carbohydrates are increased to one thousand calories, the protein limit drops to five hundred calories (125 grams).

---

188 Institute of Medicine, *Dietary Reference Intakes*, 660.
189 Ibid., 608–9.

Although the IOM hasn't set an upper limit for protein, extremely excessive protein intake increases calcium excretion in urine and can lead to calcium deficiency. In discussions of protein toxicity, there is a claim that consuming beyond four grams of protein per kilogram of one's body weight a day is unsafe.[190] It has been suggested that the cause of "rabbit starvation" is protein toxicity.[191]

Rabbit starvation refers to historic cases of people who lived for extended periods in the wilderness, surviving solely on rabbit meat, which is very lean meat. Some people theorize that the cause of death was an overdose of protein, however, the people who died in those cases had extremely low body fat, and therefore it is not known if they died from lack of dietary fat and carbohydrates or from too much protein.

HOW SHOULD PROTEIN BE COMBINED WITH OTHER FOODS?

Conventional wisdom sets adult protein-absorption limit at twenty to thirty grams per meal; what exceeds that is transformed to sugar, stored as fat, or disposed of. However, the body's protein-absorption limit is proportional to the body's muscle mass and protein needs. A one-hundred-kilogram (220 lbs.) body builder has tremendous needs; especially just after an intense workout, when the body's cells continue to absorb protein from the blood until they are satiated. A body builder would likely need at least double the protein of the average person.

Individuals have a limit of protein that they can absorb in one meal. Even a one-hundred-kilogram body builder who needs to consume two hundred grams of protein daily cannot absorb all two hundred grams in one meal and needs to spread out protein intake over several meals.

---

190   S. Bilsborough and N. Mann, "A Review of Issues of Dietary Protein Intake in Humans," *International Journal of Sport Nutrition and Exercise Metabolism* (2006), http://www.ncbi.nlm.nih.gov/pubmed/16779921.

191   Institute of Medicine, *Dietary Reference Intakes*, 693.

The protein-absorption limit can be increased in various ways:

1. **Digesting carbohydrates together with the proteins**: Hormones such as testosterone, human growth hormone, and insulin assist in the absorption of protein. Since eating carbohydrates increases insulin secretion, it increases the potential absorption of protein.
2. **Exercising before meals**: This increases the effectiveness of insulin in transferring carbohydrates and proteins from the blood into the muscles.
3. **Eating protein with fats**: This slows down the digestive process and extends protein-absorption time, enabling greater total protein absorption.

WHEN SHOULD PROTEIN BE EATEN?

Significant quantities of proteins should not be consumed shortly before or during exercise. Digestion of proteins requires a greater blood supply to be sent to the digestive tract and liver, which is impeded by exercising, since exercise draws blood to the muscles. Conversely, the digestion of proteins diminishes the supply of blood to the muscles, impeding the ability to exercise. Therefore eating a heavy meal shortly before exercising is a lose-lose situation; as both the digestive system and the muscles compete for blood supply, neither get enough blood.

Unlike proteins, free amino acids are not bound together by peptide bonds but are absorbed from the intestinal tract directly into the blood, omitting the need to process them in the intestines and liver. Therefore, many athletes take free amino acid supplements before and during exercise to minimize the breakdown of muscle protein for fuel and to speed up recovery from muscle exhaustion.

Unlike all the seventeen other amino acids, three essential amino acids (leucine, isoleucine, and valine), characterized as branched chain amino acids, or BCAAs, can be used directly as fuel by the muscles and thereby become depleted during exercise when other fuel sources are low. When stored sugar levels drop, the liver begins converting proteins and fats into sugar in the gluconeogenesis process, which uses the amino acid glutamine. As previously discussed in chapter 6, many athletes supplement with BCAAs and glutamine just before and during exercise to protect muscles from being broken down for fuel.

In summary, in respect to exercise, protein needs to be:

1. **Avoided shortly before or during exercise**: Most proteins take two to three hours to digest and absorb; therefore, if you are eating substantial amounts of proteins, ideally you should eat them at least two hours before exercising. A small amount such as ten to twenty grams or less shouldn't interfere with exercise, but the more protein you eat, the more time you need to wait before exercising.

2. **Ingested immediately afterward**: An ideal time to eat protein is immediately after exercising—especially after intense weight lifting, when the muscles are in need of protein for recovery and rebuilding. Eating carbohydrates with the proteins helps increase insulin, which aids in speeding the transfer of amino acids in the blood into the muscle cells.

DOES THE BODY STORE PROTEIN SIMILAR TO THE WAY IT STORES SUGAR AND FAT? HOW MANY TIMES PER DAY DOES ONE NEED TO EAT PROTEINS?

The common dogma is that protein can't be stored, but that is not precisely true.

The average adult male's capacity to store carbohydrates is limited to about 450 grams. Fat storage is essentially unlimited. Protein storage is perhaps more limited than carbohydrate storage; however, the bigger difference that exists between them is that there is no definitive place for the exclusive purpose of protein storage, unlike carbohydrates that is stored as glycogen in the liver and muscles.

Blood plasma, in addition to other functions, also serves as a protein reserve, containing roughly *two hundred grams* of protein in the average person. Blood plasma is the pale-yellow liquid component of blood that normally holds the blood cells in suspension in whole blood and serves to transport glucose, hormones, and so on. When body tissues become depleted of proteins, plasma proteins can act as a source of rapid replacement.

Virtually all cells in the body also have fluctuating levels of free amino acids and the ability to store and release protein. In the average adult man, it is estimated that the total free amino acids stored in the *muscle cells is over eighty-five grams*.[192] Aside from the muscle fibers, the liver stores the most amino acids and proteins.

In summary, protein is "stored" primarily in blood plasma and in the liver and muscles as free amino acids and as stored protein. However, since these proteins have multiple functions besides protein storage (e.g., blood plasma serves to maintain colloid osmotic pressure and immune system functions, transport insoluble molecules, facilitate blood coagulation, etc.), and since there are minimum levels required to maintain these other functions, it is difficult to estimate how much protein is "stored" in the average person. Therefore, without an authoritative estimate on how much protein the body usually stores as a source for replacement, I feel confident to estimate that the average adult has a protein reserve of between at least 50–150 grams, enough to survive a day or two without protein consumption without suffering the breakdown of functioning tissues as a source of protein.

Considering that normally one has sufficient protein reserves for at least one day, why is it not possible to eat protein only once per day?

---

192 J. Bergström et al., "Intracellular Free Amino Acid Concentration in Human Muscle Tissue," *Journal of Applied Physiology* (1974), http://jap.physiology.org/content/36/6/693. full.pdf.

The problem is not so much the limited storage of protein but rather the limited absorption rate. If a person consumes more protein in a meal than the body can absorb in the time that it takes to digest that meal, the excess is alternatively burned as fuel, expelled in the urine, or converted to sugar and stored as glycogen or fat. Once it is converted, it generally can't revert back to protein.

Therefore, to ensure that you absorb sufficient protein for your needs, it is recommended that you divide your protein needs between at least two to three meals. Body builders and very active people with greater protein needs should divide their protein intake between even more meals and snacks to enable their muscles to recuperate from the intensive workouts.

WHY IS IT IMPORTANT TO EAT "COMPLETE" PROTEINS?

Many food sources of proteins have incomplete proteins—proteins that lack some of the essential amino acids. When the body lacks a particular essential amino acid, its ability to synthesize many of the proteins necessary for functioning and maintaining life is limited.

Imagine writing a book without the letter *w*: you could complete a sentence here and there and maybe get in some complete paragraphs, but many sentences and paragraphs would not be able to be "synthesized," and the functionality of the book would be so compromised that it "dies."

In regard to incomplete proteins, excess amino acids in the blood are filtered by the kidneys and discarded into the urine to maintain a proper balance of amino acids for protein synthesis. When one essential amino acid is lacking, the others become proportionally too high and are not usable for protein synthesis; they are ultimately lost as proteins, either through excretion[193] or conversion to sugar for use as energy.

---

193 Guyton and Hall, *Textbook of Medical Physiology*, Saunders (2011), 833.

WHAT IS THE RDA OF ESSENTIAL AMINO ACIDS FOR ADULTS?

Measured in milligrams of amino acids per kilogram of body weight, the RDA of the essential amino acids are as follows:[194]

Leucine	42
Lysine	38
Phenylalanine + tyrosine	33
Threonine	20
Isoleucine	19
Methionine + cysteine	19
Histidine	14
Tryptophan	5
Valine	4

The total RDA of all the essential amino acids combined equals only 190 milligrams per kilogram of body weight, while RDA for *protein* equals 800 milligrams per kilogram of body weight. That is because the remaining 610 milligrams per kilogram can be a mixture of any amino acids to suffice for the body's protein homeostasis.

There are two factors that go into equating the "quality" of proteins digested: digestibility and the amount of the limiting amino acid relative to the "reference" protein (a high-quality protein). If only 50 percent of the protein is digestible or if the limiting amino acid is present in quantities less than 50 percent of the reference protein, then that item will get a low score. But remember: certain individual food items with low scores can obtain higher scores when combined with other items.

Here is the reference protein scoring pattern presented by the IOM.[195] Each amino acid is measured in milligrams per gram of protein:

---

194   Institute of Medicine, *Dietary Reference Intakes*, 680.
195   Institute of Medicine, *Dietary Reference Intakes*, 689.

Leucine	55
Lysine	51
Phenylalanine + tyrosine	47
Valine	32
Threonine	27
Isoleucine	25
Methionine + cysteine	25
Histidine	18
Tryptophan	7

The equation for measuring the protein digestibility amino acid score (PDCAAS) is: PDCAAS = mg of limiting amino acid in 1 gram of protein ÷ mg of same amino acid in 1 gram of reference protein × [% true digestibility]

WHAT FOODS CONSTITUTE A SOURCE OF "COMPLETE" PROTEIN?

Meat, fowl, fish, many dairy products, and eggs all contain substantial amounts of all the essential amino acids and are therefore referred to as complete proteins.

Vegetarian sources that have substantial amounts of all the essential amino acids are quinoa seeds, hempseed, amaranth, and chia. Soy and buckwheat have substantial amounts of nearly all the essential amino acids.

Grains and legumes on their own lack certain essential amino acids (and are therefore referred to as incomplete proteins); however, they complement each other when combined, providing all the essential amino acids.

Most commonly, the limiting amino acids are lysine, threonine, tryptophan, and sulfur-containing amino acids. Animal products are the highest sources of lysine and threonine, and nuts and seeds are the highest sources of tryptophan and sulfur-containing amino acids, hence the importance of having a balanced diet.

WHAT FOODS ARE RICH IN PROTEIN?

Following is the percentage of protein of different foods by weight:

Whey and soy protein isolate*	90%
Meats, fowl, fish, legumes, and certain dairy products	30–50%
Seeds and nuts	15–20%
Grains and eggs	10–15%
Fruits and vegetables	0–3%

Avoid or limit powders that use artificial sweeteners such as aspartame and sucralose—the preferred sweeteners are stevia and sugar alcohols.

HOW MUCH PROTEIN IS IDEAL?

According to the IOM, the RDAs for the division of macronutrients (according to the percentage of total caloric intake) are as follows:

Carbohydrates	45–65%
Fats	20–35%
Proteins	10–35%

According to Dr. Sears, in the Zone diet, the division should be as follows:

Carbohydrates	40%
Fats	30%
Proteins	30%

For people with high blood sugar and hyperinsulinemia who need to minimize carbohydrate intake to stabilize blood sugar levels, the Zone division is better because it sets a lower limit for carbohydrates and a higher base requirement for proteins. As mentioned earlier, the RDA minimum for proteins is disputed, as it can lead to deficiencies.

For people with extremely high blood sugar and instability, even less than 40 percent carbohydrates is recommended, requiring an even higher percentage of the intake of proteins and fats. Numerous studies demonstrate that high protein diets are more satiating than high fats or carbohydrates and more conducive to reducing caloric intake and losing weight.[196, 197, 198]

196   Arne Astrup, "The Satiating Power of Protein: A Key to Obesity Prevention?" *American Journal of Clinical Nutrition* (2005), http://ajcn.nutrition.org/content/82/1/1.full.

197   H. J. Leidy et al., "The Effects of Consuming Frequent, Higher Protein Meals on Appetite and Satiety During Weight Loss in Overweight/Obese Men," *Obesity* (2011), http://www.ncbi.nlm.nih.gov/pubmed/20847729

198   T. L. Halton and F. B. Hu, "The Effects of High Protein Diets on Thermogenesis, Satiety and Weight Loss: A Critical Review," *Journal of the American College of Nutrition* (2004), http://www.colorado.edu/intphys/Class/IPHY3700_Greene/pdfs/discussionEssay/thermogenesisSatiety/HaltonProtein2004.pdf.

12

Carbohydrates: Sugar, Starch, and Fiber

One of the four primary elements for alleviating the metabolic syndrome is limiting the glycemic load of meals by reducing carbohydrates. Since fiber is a type of carbohydrate, by reducing carbohydrates, one is likely to get less dietary fiber. However, most people get less than half the RDA of fiber—a type of carbohydrate—even though they are consuming too many carbohydrates. This chapter explains the crucial benefits of fiber and includes tables listing the fiber content of various foods to enable you to formulate a well-planned diet, attaining sufficient fiber even with reduced carbohydrates. This chapter explains the following:

- The Caloric Difference between Sugar, Starch, Soluble Fiber, and Insoluble Fiber
- The Functions of Carbohydrates
- Recommended Amount of Carbohydrate Intake as a Percentage of Total Caloric Intake
- The Health Benefits of Fiber
- Food Sources High in Fiber

APPENDIX TO CHAPTER 12
- The Different Structures and the Different Physiological Effects of Sugars, Starches, and Fiber
- Types of Sugars and Starches

TYPES OF CARBOHYDRATES AND THE CALORIC DIFFERENCE BETWEEN SUGAR, STARCH, AND FIBER

The American Diabetes Association divides carbohydrates into three categories:

- Sugars
- Starches
- Fibers

All carbohydrates have stored energy—4.1 calories per gram, to be exact—however, for humans, fiber *contributes* fewer calories than sugars and starches because it cannot be fully absorbed by the body. Sugars and starches do provide 4.1 calories per gram, as the human body has specific enzymes to break them down into glucose, fructose, and galactose, which can then be absorbed by the body. But the human body lacks enzymes to break down fiber. Insoluble fiber does not change inside the body, so the body cannot absorb it, and it provides no energy.

Soluble fiber is the edible parts of plants or similar carbohydrates. What is unique to soluble fiber is that it is very resistant to digestion and absorption in the human small intestine, with complete or partial fermentation in the large intestine. Partially fermented by bacteria in the large intestine, soluble fiber contributes some energy when broken down and absorbed. Dietitians have not reached a consensus on how much energy is actually absorbed, but most estimates approximate two calories per gram.

In some countries, fiber is not listed on nutrition labels and is considered as though it provides no energy. In other countries, all fiber must be listed and is simplistically considered as providing 4.1 calories per gram. According to US law, soluble fiber must be counted as four calories per gram, but insoluble fiber may be (and usually is) treated as not providing energy and is not mentioned on the label.

In round figures:

- Sugar and starch = four calories per gram
- Soluble fiber = two calories per gram
- Insoluble fiber = zero calories per gram

SUGAR AND STARCH: THE BODY'S PRIMARY SOURCES OF ENERGY

Relative to fats and proteins, sugars and starches are broken down into glucose quickly and as such serve as the body's primary source of energy. All body cells require glucose, the simplest form of carbohydrate, so they can produce ATP (adenosine triphosphate—intercellular fuel) and properly function.

When glucose is not consumed in the diet, the body converts fats and proteins into glucose. Also, certain amino acids and fatty acids can be burned as an alternative fuel to glucose.

FIBROUS POLYSACCHARIDES

Dietary fiber is the edible parts of plants or analogous carbohydrates that are resistant to digestion and absorption in the human small intestine, with complete or partial fermentation in the large intestine. It includes polysaccharides, oligosaccharides, lignin, and associated plant substances. Dietary fiber promotes beneficial physiologic effects, including laxation, blood cholesterol reduction, and/or blood glucose reduction.

There are many dozens of polysaccharides. Here are detailed only two: cellulose, because it is the most common, and inulin, because it is so beneficial and useful.

- **Cellulose**: A structural constituent of the cell walls of plants, cellulose is the most common type of polysaccharide on earth. This rigid insoluble carbohydrate can only be digested by herbivores such as cows, sheep, horses, and the like, as these animals have enzyme systems and bacteria in their stomachs that can break down cellulose. Humans do not have these enzymes, and therefore cellulose passes through the digestive tract unchanged.

- **Inulin**: A soluble polysaccharide, inulin is typically extracted by manufacturers from enriched plant sources such as chicory roots or Jerusalem artichokes for use in prepared foods. Subtly sweet, it can be used to replace sugar, fat, and flour. It is often used to improve the flow and mixing qualities of powdered nutritional supplements, and it has significant potential health value as a prebiotic fermentable fiber (prebiotics are chemicals that induce the growth or activity of microorganisms that contribute to the well-being of their hosts).

Inulin is advantageous because it is low in calories, typically containing about one calorie per gram. As a prebiotic fermentable fiber, its metabolism by gut flora yields short-chain fatty acids, which increase absorption of calcium,[199] magnesium,[200] and iron, resulting from the up-regulation (increase) of mineral-transporting genes and their membrane-transport proteins within the colon wall.[201] Additionally, inulin promotes an increase in the mass and health of intestinal *Lactobacillus* and *Bifidobacterium* populations.

HEALTH BENEFITS OF FIBER

According to the *Dietary Guidelines for Americans 2010*, produced by the US Department of Health and Human Services, dietary fiber may help reduce the risk of cardiovascular disease, obesity, and type 2 diabetes.

---

199 S. A. Abrams et al., "A Combination of Prebiotic Short- and Long-Chain Inulin-Type Fructans Enhances Calcium Absorption and Bone Mineralization in Young Adolescents," *American Journal of Clinical Nutrition* (2005), http://www.ncbi.nlm.nih.gov/pubmed/16087995.

200 C. Coudray, C. Demigné, and Y. Rayssiguier, "Effects of Dietary Fibers on Magnesium Absorption in Animals and Humans," *Journal of Nutrition* (2003), http://www.ncbi.nlm.nih.gov/pubmed/12514257.

201 E. Tako et al., "Dietary Inulin Affects the Expression of Intestinal Enterocyte Iron Transporters, Receptors and Storage Protein and Alters the Microbiota in the Pig Intestine," *British Journal of Nutrition* (2008), http://www.ncbi.nlm.nih.gov/pubmed/17868492.

Here are some of the ways that consuming fiber prevents these conditions as well as some of its other benefits:

- **Removes cholesterol**: *Soluble fiber* binds bile acids, which are digestive liquids made from cholesterol. Consuming a high-fiber diet leads to increased excretion of bile acids and thus increased removal of cholesterol from the body, lowering LDL ("bad") cholesterol and reducing the risk of cardiovascular disease.

- **Produces healthful compounds**: During the fermentation of *soluble fiber*, healthful compounds, such as prebiotics, are produced, increasing the absorption of valuable minerals.[202, 203, 204]

- **Slows absorption of sugar and stabilizes blood sugar**: *Soluble fiber* attracts water and forms a viscous gel during digestion, slowing the emptying of the stomach and intestinal transit, shielding carbohydrates from enzymes, and delaying the absorption of glucose, which lowers variance in blood sugar levels.[205, 206, 207, 208]

- **Maintains the health of the digestive tract**: *Insoluble fiber* binds water as it travels through the digestive tract. This helps

---

202 K. E. Scholz-Ahrens and J. Schrezenmeir, "Inulin and Oligofructose and Mineral Metabolism: The Evidence from Animal Trials," *Journal of Nutrition* (2007), http://www.ncbi.nlm.nih.gov/pubmed/17951495.

203 J. L. Greger, "Nondigestible Carbohydrates and Mineral Bioavailability," *Journal of Nutrition* (1999), http://jn.nutrition.org/content/129/7/1434S.full.

204 Ladislav Raschkaand and Daniel Hannelore, "Mechanisms Underlying the Effects of Inulin-Type Fructans on Calcium Absorption in the Large Intestine of Rats," *Bone* 37, no. 5 (November 2005): 728–35, http://www.thebonejournal.com/article/S8756-3282(05)00249-8/abstract.

205 D. J. Jenkins et al., "Dietary Fibres, Fibre Analogues, and Glucose Tolerance: Importance of Viscosity," *British Medical Journal*, (1978), http://www.bmj.com/content/1/6124/1392.

206 Institute of Medicine, *Dietary Reference Intakes*, 380–82.

207 Sareen S. Gropper, Jack L. Smith, and James L. Groff, *Advanced Nutrition and Human Metabolism*, 5th edition, Cengage Learning (2008), 114.

208 C. A. Edwards, I. T. Johnson, and N. W. Read, "Do Viscous Polysaccharides Slow Absorption by Inhibiting Diffusion or Convection?" *European Journal of Clinical Nutrition* (April 1988), http://www.ncbi.nlm.nih.gov/pubmed/2840277.

make stools softer and bulkier and helps prevent colon diseases, colon cancer, constipation, hemorrhoids, and diverticulitis. (Diverticulitis, an inflammation of the intestine, is one of the most common age-related disorders of the colon in Western society.)

- **Increases insulin sensitivity**: Resistant starch, a type of *insoluble fiber*, has been shown to directly increase insulin sensitivity when eaten together with caloric carbohydrates,[209, 210, 211] contributing to reduced risk of type 2 diabetes.

- **Reduces appetite**: Fiber makes us feel full sooner and stays in our stomach longer than other substances that we eat, slowing down our rate of digestion and keeping us feeling full longer.

- **Reduces fat absorption**: Fiber also moves fat through our digestive system faster so that less fat is absorbed.

- **Lowers intestinal pH**: Lowering the pH protects the intestinal lining from formation of colonic polyps and increases absorption of dietary minerals.[212]

HOW AND WHY TO GET MORE DIETARY FIBER

*The average American consumes less than half of the minimum RDA of fiber recommended by the FDA:[213] **fourteen grams of fiber per one thousand calories consumed (or 1.4 grams for every 100 calories).***

209 M. D. Robertson et al., "Prior Short-Term Consumption of Resistant Starch Enhances Postprandial Insulin Sensitivity in Healthy Subjects," *Diabetologia* 46, no. 5 (May 2003), 659–65, http://link.springer.com/article/10.1007%2Fs00125-003-1081-0.

210 W. Q. Zhang et al., "Effects of Resistant Starch on Insulin Resistance of Type 2 Diabetes Mellitus Patients," *Zhonghua Yu Fang Yi Xue Za Zhi* (2007), http://www.ncbi.nlm.nih.gov/pubmed/17605234.

211 K. L. Johnston et al., "Resistant Starch Improves Insulin Sensitivity in Metabolic Syndrome," *Diabetic Medicine* (2010), http://www.ncbi.nlm.nih.gov/pubmed/20536509.

212 J. L. Greger, "Nondigestible Carbohydrates and Mineral Bioavailability," *Journal of Nutrition* (1999), http://jn.nutrition.org/content/129/7/1434S.full.

213 Institute of Medicine, *Dietary Reference Intakes*, 339.

Some calories we consume don't have any fiber, such as meat, fish, eggs, and dairy. So we need to compensate by eating foods high in fiber. Since the RDA of fiber is 1.4 grams per one hundred calories, we need to seek out foods that are at least double that—2.8 grams per one hundred calories—to compensate for the foods we eat that don't have any fiber. You can find foods high in fiber in the list below.

The best way to obtain dietary fiber is to eat foods such as vegetables, whole grains, legumes, fruits, seeds, and nuts. Refined grains have had most of their fiber removed.

FIBER CONTENTS IN FOOD

Fiber supplements are available to increase the intake of dietary fiber; however, most experts recommend that fiber should be obtained through the consumption of foods, because food sources enable you to consume many micronutrients and bioactive compounds contained in high-fiber foods, which provide their own nutritional benefits.

Dietary fiber is found in the following foods in descending order of its concentration (per calories):

- Vegetables, whole grains, and legumes (3–12 g fiber/100 cal)
- Fruits (3–6 g fiber/100 cal)
- Seeds (1–7 g fiber/100 cal)
- Nuts (1–2 g fiber/100 cal)
- Refined grains (0.5–2 g fiber/100 cal)

Keep in mind that most adults need to digest at least thirty to fifty grams of fiber daily, or fourteen grams for every one thousand calories.

GRAMS OF FIBER IN FOOD GROUPS PER CALORIES

The following tables are derived from the US Department of Agriculture's National Nutrient Database. For the purposes of practicality, I have chosen only a select group of the thousands of items listed by the USDA. Additionally, the department only lists fiber and calories per one hundred grams, whereas my unique calculations of fiber per one hundred calories (based on the department's information) are more useful. And although the original list places the items in alphabetical order, I have ordered my list according to fiber concentration to present a more coherent picture.

The tables put facts into surprising perspective, such as mushrooms being substantially higher in fiber than carrots (per calorie) and green beans having more than double the fiber of onions and quadruple the fiber of corn.[214]

Vegetables are very high in fiber per calorie; however, they are low in fiber in proportion to their weight. Therefore, unless one eats huge amounts of vegetables, one will need to get the RDA of fiber from other sources as well. Table 12-1 shows a list of various vegetables and their amount of fiber per one hundred calories.

TABLE 12-1. Amount of fiber in vegetables per calorie

Vegetable (1–3% fiber by weight)	3–12 g fiber/100cal
Artichokes	16.9
Dry seaweed	14.0
Romaine lettuce	12.3
Cabbage	12.1
Green beans	10.7
Spinach	9.6

214 If you have a favorite food item that is not listed here, you can get the information on the USDA's site: "Nutritional Nutrient Database for Standard Reference Release 27," US Department of Agriculture, http://ndb.nal.usda.gov/ndb/nutrients/report/nutrientsfrm?m ax=25&offset=0&totCount=0&nutrient1=291&nutrient2=&nutrient3=&subset=0&fg=20 &sort=f&measureby=g.

TABLE 12-1. Continued

Vegetable	fiber/100cal
Broccoli	9.4
Asparagus	9.0
Celery	8.9
Mushrooms	8.7
Iceberg lettuce	8.6
Sweet green peppers	8.5
Eggplant	7.4
Squash	7.0
Carrots	6.8
Sweet red peppers	6.8
Green peas	6.3
Tomatoes	5.0
Cooked beets	4.5
Cucumber	4.3
Onions	4.2
Cooked sweet potato	3.3
Corn	2.8
Baked potatoes w/skin	2.4

Note: All figures are based on information provided by the US
Department of Agriculture.

Whole grains and legumes have less fiber per calorie than most vegetables; however, since they are much denser in fiber in proportion to their weight, you can easily reach your RDA of fiber by eating two meals a day of reasonably sized portions of whole grains and/or legumes. Additionally, a large percentage of the calories in grains and legumes are proteins as opposed to the calories in fruits and vegetables that are nearly all sugar or starch calories with little to no protein. Table 12-2 shows a list of whole grains and legumes and their corresponding amount of fiber per one hundred calories.

TABLE 12-2. Grams of fiber in whole grains and legumes per 100 calories

WHOLE GRAIN (8–16% FIBER/WEIGHT)	3–7 G FIBER/100 CAL
Crude corn bran	35.2
Crude wheat bran	19.8
Dark rye flour	7.3
Crude rice bran	6.6
Raw oat bran	6.2
Raw barley	4.4
Rye grain	4.4
Whole-grain wheat flour	3.1
Raw spelt	3.1
Cooked spelt	3.1
Buckwheat (cooked)	2.9
Buckwheat (raw)	2.9
Oats	2.7
Instant oat cereal boiled w/water	2.4

LEGUME (COOKED) (6–9 PERCENT FIBER/WEIGHT)	4–7 G FIBER/100 CAL
French beans (cooked)	7.3
Lentils (cooked)	6.9
Black beans (cooked)	6.6
Pinto beans (cooked)	6.3
White beans (cooked)	6.1
Lima beans (cooked)	6.1
Kidney beans (cooked)	5.0
Chick peas (cooked)	4.6
Soybeans (cooked)	3.6
Raw/roasted peanuts	1.5
Peanut butter	1.4

Note: All figures are based on information provided by the US Department of Agriculture.

In general, most fruits are not especially high when measured in grams of fiber per calorie. When measured by weight, most fruits are relatively low in fiber, and as such, people need to get the bulk of their RDA of fiber from other sources.

TABLE 12-3. Grams of fiber in fruits per 100 calories

FRUIT (1/2–3% FIBER/WEIGHT)	3–6 G FIBER/100 CAL
Blackberries	12.3
Strawberries	6.2
Pears	5.4
Oranges	5.2
Kiwi	4.9
Apples w/skin	4.6
Avocados	4.2
Blueberries	4.2
Apricots	4.1
Dried figs	3.9
Raw figs	3.9
Peaches	3.8
Grapefruit	3.4
Sweet cherries	3.3
Sour cherries	3.2
Melon	3.2
Plums	3.0
Bananas	2.9
Pineapple	2.8
Dates	2.7
Mangos	2.7
Apples w/o skin	2.7
Olives	2.3
Raisins	1.3
Grapes	1.3
Watermelon	1.3

Note: All figures are based on information provided by the US Department of Agriculture.

Both chia seeds and ground flaxseed are very high in the essential fatty acid omega-3. They are also very high in important vitamins and minerals as well as fiber. However, eat them sparingly, because eating just one hundred grams of them will load you up with approximately five hundred calories! While nuts are also nutritious, their nutritional value doesn't compare to chia and flaxseed, yet they are just as high in calories.

TABLE 12-4. Amount of fiber in seeds and nuts per calories

SEEDS (10–20% FIBER/WEIGHT)	1–7 G FIBER/100 CAL
Dried chia seeds	7.1
Flaxseed	5.1
Roasted pumpkin seeds	4.1
Roasted sesame seeds	2.5
Dry-roasted sunflower seeds	1.6
Pumpkin seed	1.1

NUTS (7–12% FIBER/WEIGHT)	1–2 G FIBER/100 CAL
Almonds	2.2
Pistachios	1.8
Hazelnuts	1.5
Pecans	1.4
Macadamia Nuts	1.2
Walnuts	1.0
Cashews	0.6

Note: All figures are based on information provided by the US Department of Agriculture.

Refined grains have little fiber or other nutritional value per calorie.

TABLE 12-5. Amount of fiber in refined grains per calories

Refined Grains (1–4% fiber/weight)	½–2 g fiber/100 cal
Macaroni (whole-wheat, cooked)	2.2
Light rye flour	2.2
Cornmeal, whole-grain, white	2.0
Corn flour	1.8
Rice (brown, cooked)	1.6
Millet (cooked)	1.1
Noodles (egg, cooked)	0.9
Millet flour	0.9
White wheat flour	0.7
Raw white rice	0.4

Note: All figures are based on information provided by the US Department of Agriculture.

The following tables repeat the information in the former tables, with foods listed in order of fiber concentration by *weight*, as opposed to the previous list that orders the items by fiber concentration per *calorie*.

PERCENTAGE OF FIBER BY WEIGHT

TABLE 12-6. Percentage of fiber in seeds by weight

Seed	10–20% fiber/weight
Dried chia seeds	34.4
Flaxseed	27.3
Roasted pumpkin seeds	18.4
Roasted sesame seeds	14.0
Dry roasted sunflower seeds	9.0
Pumpkin seed	6.5

TABLE 12-7. Percentage of fiber in whole grains by weight

Whole grain	8–16% fiber/weight
Crude corn bran	79
Crude wheat bran	42.8
Dark rye flour	23.8
Crude rice bran	21
Barley (raw)	15.6
Oat bran (raw)	15.4
Rye grain	15.1
Whole-grain wheat flour	10.7
Spelt (raw)	10.7
Oats	10.6
Buckwheat (raw)	10
Millet (raw)	8.5
Light rye flour	8
Cornmeal (whole grain, white)	7.3
Corn flour	6.4
Brown rice (raw)	3.4
Instant oat cereal boiled w/water	1.7

Note: All figures are based on information provided by the US Department of Agriculture.

TABLE 12-8. Percentage of fiber in nuts and legumes by weight

Nut	7–12% fiber/weight
Almonds	12.5
Pistachios	10.3
Hazelnuts	9.7
Pecans	9.6
Macadamia nuts	8.6
Walnuts	6.7
Cashews	3.3

LEGUMES (COOKED)	6–9% FIBER/WEIGHT
Soy flour	17.5
French beans (cooked)	9.4
Pinto beans (cooked)	9.0
Black beans (cooked)	8.7
White beans (cooked)	8.5
Peanuts (raw/roasted)	8.5
Peanut butter	8.0
Lentils (cooked)	7.9
Chickpeas (cooked)	7.6
Lima beans (cooked)	7.0
Kidney beans (cooked)	6.4
Soybeans (cooked)	6.0

Note: All figures are based on information provided by the US Department of Agriculture.

TABLE 12-9. Percentage of fiber in refined grains by weight

REFINED GRAIN	1–4% FIBER/WEIGHT
Spelt (cooked)	3.9
Millet flour	3.5
Brown rice (raw)	3.5
Macaroni (whole wheat, cooked)	2.8
Flour (white wheat)	2.7
Buckwheat (cooked)	2.7
Rice (brown, cooked)	1.8
Rice (raw, white)	1.4
Millet (cooked)	1.3
Noodles (egg, cooked)	1.2

Note: All figures are based on information provided by the US Department of Agriculture.

TABLE 12-10. Percentage of fiber in vegetables by weight

Vegetable	1–3% fiber/weight
Dry seaweed	36.7
Artichokes	8.6
Green peas	5.1
Broccoli	3.3
Green beans	3.0
Carrots	2.8
Corn	2.7
Mushrooms	2.7
Eggplant	2.5
Cooked sweet potato	2.5
Baked potatoes w/skin	2.2
Spinach	2.2
Romaine lettuce	2.1
Sweet red peppers	2.1
Cooked beets	2.0
Asparagus	2.0
Onions	1.7
Celery	1.6
Sweet green peppers	1.7
Cabbage	1.7
Squash	1.4
Iceberg lettuce	1.2
Tomatoes	1.0
Cucumber	0.6

Note: All figures are based on information provided by the US Department of Agriculture.

TABLE 12-11. Percentage of fiber in fruits by weight

Fruits	1/2–3% fiber/weight
Dried figs	9.8
Dates	7.5
Avocados	6.7
Blackberries	5.3
Raisins	4.0
Olives	3.3
Pears	3.1
Kiwi	3.0
Raw figs	2.9
Bananas	2.6
Apples w/skin	2.4
Oranges	2.4
Blueberries	2.4
Sweet cherries	2.1
Strawberries	2.0
Apricots	2.0
Sour cherries	1.6
Mangos	1.6
Peaches	1.5
Plums	1.4
Pineapple	1.4
Apples w/o skin	1.3
Grapefruit	1.1
Grapes	0.9
Melon	0.9
Watermelon	0.4

Note: All figures are based on information provided by the US Department of Agriculture.

Appendix to Chapter 12

The Different Structure and Different Physiological Effects of Sugars, Starches, and Fiber

The purpose of this brief appendix is to provide some clarity and understanding concerning different types of carbohydrates.

The general composition of carbohydrates is CH_2O (C = Carbon, H = Hydrogen, O = Oxygen). The amount of each atom varies between the different types of carbohydrates. In most cases, the hydrogen-to-oxygen ratio is two to one.

SUGARS AND STARCHES

Carbohydrates, also known as *saccharides*, are classified according to the number of single-carbohydrate molecules in each chemical structure. Carbohydrate compounds having just one carbohydrate molecule are called *monosaccharides*. Compounds with two carbohydrate molecules are called *disaccharides*, and compounds containing at least three (sometimes as many as sixty thousand) carbohydrate molecules are named *polysaccharides*. All carbohydrates are either monosaccharides or can be hydrolyzed (broken down) into monosaccharides.

Sugars—monosaccharides and disaccharides—are referred to as *simple carbs*, since their simple structures allow the body to quickly break them down.

Starches—polysaccharides—are referred to as *complex carbohydrates* and take longer to break down due to their more sophisticated structures.

Polysaccharides include starch, dextrin, glycogen, and numerous types of soluble and insoluble fiber.

Monosaccharaides and Disaccharides

Monosaccharaides and disaccharides are types of sugars. They are water soluble, crystalline in structure, and sweet tasting, and their names all end in the suffix *–ose*, meaning sugar.

Glucose, Fructose, and Galactose

The three main examples of monosaccharaides are glucose, fructose, and galactose. Glucose, also known as blood sugar (and dextrose or grape sugar), is absorbed into the bloodstream from the small intestine. Insulin speeds its transport into muscles, the liver, and other cells, which use the glucose to generate ATP, the body's energy molecule, through the metabolic process known as glycolysis. Quantities of glucose that are in excess of the body's immediate needs are either stored as glycogen in muscle and liver or converted into fatty acids.

Unlike glucose, fructose and galactose are generally not *directly* used for energy production and are less subjected to regulation by insulin. They are primarily broken down in the liver, producing intermediates used in glycolysis en route to generating new ATP molecules. Galactose is metabolized also in the brain and is therefore known as brain sugar; in infants, it is metabolized to develop the brain, and in adults it is used to synthesize the amino acids glutamate and glutamine.

Sucrose, Lactose, and Maltose

The three most common disaccharides are sucrose, lactose, and maltose. Sucrose, or table sugar, consists of a glucose molecule bonded to a fructose molecule. It is broken down in the small intestine by the enzyme sucrase, which splits up the two molecules.

Lactose (milk sugar) is made up of a glucose and galactose molecule. The enzyme lactase, present in the small intestine, separates those two molecules. In the absence of lactase, the lactose is not digested in the small intestine. Rather it enters the large intestine, where the bacteria digest the lactose, causing gas production. A person with a lactase deficiency is said to be "lactose intolerant."

Maltose (malt sugar) contains two glucose molecules that are bonded together. The two glucose molecules are split up by the enzyme maltase inside the small intestine.

Nonfibrous Polysaccharides

Nonfibrous polysaccharides consist of starch, dextrin, and glycogen, which have the following properties:

- **Starches**: Most starches are a mix of amylose and amylopectin, the proportion varying according to the type of plant.
- **Dextrins**: These are formed from starch either through cooking or digestion; when broken down (hydrolyzed), they render maltose.
- **Glycogen**: The body stores carbohydrates in the form of glycogen. About two-thirds of glycogen reserves are stored in the muscle and one-third in the liver.

Fats

The fourth primary element for alleviating the metabolic syndrome is measured glycemic load. For most people, a measured glycemic load includes a reduction in carbohydrates and limiting high GI carbohydrates. A reduction in carbohydrates needs to be balanced by an increase in fats and/or proteins. But not all fats are equal; some are advantageous to get more of, and others should be avoided. This chapter explains the following:

- The Biological Functions of Fats
- Nine-Point Summary of How Much Fat to Eat and What Types
- In-Depth Analysis of Three Categories of Fat: Beneficial, Essential, and Detrimental
- Understanding Blood Test Cholesterol Levels: HDL, LDL, and Triglyceride Levels
- How to Reduce LDL Levels
- Appendix: Understanding the Terms *Saturated*, *Unsaturated*, *Polyunsaturated*, *Cis*, and *Trans*

THE BIOLOGICAL FUNCTIONS OF FATS

Fats are a major source of energy, providing nine calories per gram in comparison to carbohydrates and proteins, which provide just four calories per gram.

Incorporating fats into one's meal slows digestion and triggers responses in the brain, yielding a sense of satiation and curbing appetite. Fats provide longer-lasting energy than carbohydrates and proteins and enable energy intake without spiking blood sugar levels and their ill effects.

Beyond the energy fats provide, they have the following essential functions:

1. To assist with growth and development
2. To aid in absorption of fat-soluble vitamins A, D, E, and K, and carotenoids (plant pigments, which the body converts into vitamin A; they are healthy antioxidants and enhance immune response to infections)
3. To serve as building blocks for cell membranes
4. To serve as building blocks for hormones and intracellular messenger molecules
5. To serve as building blocks for bile acids (needed for digestion and metabolism of fats, as well as maintaining cholesterol homeostasis)
6. To act on DNA (activating or inhibiting transcription factors)
7. To aid in the growth of intestinal bacteria, which help produce B vitamins
8. To aid in mental focus and cognitive function
9. To insulate the body from cold
10. To pad and protect nerves and organs
11. To play a role in blood coagulation, brain development, and the regulation of inflammation in the body
12. To serve as cellular barriers, regulating the type of substances that enter and leave cells
13. To give structure to lipoproteins—a family of proteins that help transport fatty compounds like cholesterol throughout the bloodstream
14. To help maintain skin, hair, and liver health, memory, and vision
15. To serve in transport and metabolism of fatty acids in and out of mitochondria (structures inside cells that utilize glucose, fatty acids, and some amino acids combined with oxygen to generate ATP, the body's cellular fuel)

NINE-POINT SUMMARY OF HOW MUCH FAT TO EAT AND WHAT TYPES

Nine essential points about the findings on fat, the most important types to eat, and the best types of food to find them in are listed below.

1. According to the US Department of Agriculture, an acceptable macronutrient distribution range for total fat is 20 to 35 percent of energy (total caloric intake). Those who choose low-carbohydrate diets must meet their energy needs primarily from proteins and fats, thus needing a fat consumption of at least 30 percent of caloric intake.

2. The most important fats/oils to include in the diet are EPA/DHA fatty acids (two types of omega-3), found in *fish oil*. Consuming at least two portions of fish per week is recommended.

3. The next-most-important oil, ALA fatty acids (the third type of omega-3), is found in *ground flaxseed* and in *chia seed*. Eating a heaping tablespoon of each every day, perhaps along with a handful of nuts or seeds, is excellent.

4. Use canola and olive oil for cooking and salads, as they are low in saturated and omega-6 fatty acids and high in monounsaturated and omega-3 fatty acids.

5. Choose healthy meat and dairy sources. These include cottage cheese, healthy cultured yogurt, skim milk, and lean meats. Grass-fed meat and dairy products have three to five times the amount of the beneficial conjugated linoleic acid; choose grass fed when possible. See our website idealmetabolism.com to locate where to buy the best quality grass-fed meat and dairy products.

6. Limit sources high in omega-6 fatty acids, such as soybeans, and sunflower, corn, soybean, and cottonseed oils.

7. Limit sources high in saturated fats, such as palm oil, fatty dairy, and meat products.

8. Minimize sources high in cholesterol such as egg yolks, animal organs, butter, whipped cream, cream cheese, and other fatty

cheeses, and limit sources of moderate levels of cholesterol, such as meat, poultry, fish, and other dairy products.

9. Avoid trans fats like the plague. Consider the following:

   a. Commercially fried foods are usually made with shortening or partially hydrogenated vegetable oils. Avoid them.

   b. Partially hydrogenated oils are trans fats. If trans fats are listed on the label on a commercial snack food, avoid it.

   c. Commercially baked foods such as doughnuts, frozen pizza, cookies, crackers, muffins, pies, and cakes usually contain trans fats. Avoid them.

   d. Substitute soft margarines (liquid or tub varieties) instead of harder stick forms. Look for "Zero grams trans fat" on the nutrition facts label and for "No hydrogenated oils" in the ingredients list.

In-Depth Analysis of Three Categories of Fat: Beneficial, Essential, and Detrimental There are so many names of different types of fats that it's confusing. There are saturated, monounsaturated, polyunsaturated, trans, cis, omega-3, omega-6, omega-9, triacylglycerol, glycerol, phospholipids, sterols, EPA, DHA, ALA, LDL cholesterol, HDL cholesterol, and more. This chapter explains these terms in a simple and organized fashion, making them easier to remember. Ultimately it is important to know the meaning of each of these terms so that we can distinguish between the healthy and unhealthy fats that we choose to ingest.

For practicality, I have categorized fats into three groups: *beneficial*, those we can eat; *essential*, those we need to should eat or should eat more of; and *detrimental*, those we need to avoid.

Beneficial Fats

Most types of fats have known benefits to human health, such as the benefits listed above. However, most types are nonessential, since the body produces these fats according to its needs from other macronutrients.

There is one particular nonessential fat, CLA (conjugated linoleic acid), that is more important to obtain than other beneficial fats for two reasons—one reason being that in our modern era, CLA is hardly available in the marketplace and is sorely lacking in our diets. Another reason is because it is very helpful in losing weight because it suppresses appetite, increases energy expenditure, decreases lipogenesis (the transformation of blood sugar into body fat), increases lipolysis (breakdown of body fat), and speeds up apoptosis (destruction) of fat cells.[215, 216, 217, 218] Additionally, CLA is known to add muscle[219] and lower the risk of diabetes[220] and cancer.[221]

Personally, I suspect that the lack of CLA in our modern era is a significant contributor to the epidemics of obesity and diabetes. CLA is found in significant quantities in meat and dairy products in which the animals fed on grass. Today, cows are fattened up with cheap grains, as that is the most cost-effective method for farmers to get the most pounds and gallons of meat and milk. In the old days, cows grazed on grass and were leaner. Grass-fed cows' meat and milk has three to five

215 Arion Kennedy et al., "Antiobesity Mechanisms of Action of Conjugated Linoleic Acid," *Journal of Nutritional Biochemistry*, (December 2009), http://www.ncbi.nlm.nih.gov/pmc/articles/PMC2826589/.

216 A. C. Watras et al., "The Role of Conjugated Linoleic Acid in Reducing Body Fat and Preventing Holiday Weight Gain," *International Journal of Obesity*, (March 2007), http://www.ncbi.nlm.nih.gov/pubmed/16924272.

217 S. C. Chen et al., "Effect of Conjugated Linoleic Acid Supplementation on Weight Loss and Body Fat Composition in a Chinese Population," *Nutrition*, (May 2012), http://www.ncbi.nlm.nih.gov/pubmed/22261578.

218 Henrietta Blankson et al., "Conjugated Linoleic Acid Reduces Body Fat Mass in Overweight and Obese Humans," *Journal of Nutrition*, (June 2000), http://jn.nutrition.org/content/130/12/2943.short.

219 S. E. Steck et al., "Conjugated Linoleic Acid Supplementation for Twelve Weeks Increases Lean Body Mass in Obese Humans," *Journal of Nutrition*, (May 2007), http://www.ncbi.nlm.nih.gov/pubmed/17449580.

220 N. Castro-Webb, E. A. Ruiz-Narváez, and H. Campos, "Cross-Sectional Study of Conjugated Linoleic Acid in Adipose Tissue and Risk of Diabetes," *American Journal of Clinical Nutrition*, (July 1996), http://www.ncbi.nlm.nih.gov/pubmed/22648724.

221 A. Białek and A. Tokarz, "Conjugated Linoleic Acid as a Potential Protective Factor in Prevention of Breast Cancer," *Postępy higieny i medycyny doświadczalnej*, (January 2013), http://www.ncbi.nlm.nih.gov/pubmed/23475478

times more CLA than products from grain-fed animals and has much less saturated fat.

Because of its significant benefits, CLA supplements have become the rage. However, there are twenty-eight types of conjugated linoleic acids (CLAs), and those manufactured and sold as supplements are unhealthy, harmful, artificially produced trans fats, not sharing the biological benefits of naturally occurring CLAs in meat and milk. Studies with CLA supplements have shown some benefits for animals but rarely demonstrated any benefits for humans.

According to one study, the most effective dosage for human adults is roughly three and a half grams of CLA per day, while more than that adds no additional benefits. [222] Dosage in this context is referring to natural CLA found in food as opposed to manufactured supplements. A ten-ounce portion (roughly three hundred grams) of grass-fed beef contains about three and a half grams of CLA.

See our website idealmetabolism.com for updated information detailing where to buy the best quality grass-fed meat and milk products.

Essential Fats

It is essential to obtain omega-3 and omega-6 fatty acids from the diet, as the body cannot produce these on its own. These fatty acids enable the body to reduce the risk of chronic heart conditions and cancer;[223] improve memory and concentration; relieve depression; and reduce inflammation, arthritis, and asthma.

It is rare to be deficient in omega-6 fatty acids, as sources rich in omega-6 include most vegetable oils, poultry, grains, nuts, and seeds. In fact, according to several studies,[224] modern Western diets have exces-

---

222 Henrietta Blankson et al., "Conjugated Linoleic Acid Reduces Body Fat Mass in Overweight and Obese Humans," *Journal of Nutrition*, (June 2000), http://jn.nutrition.org/content/130/12/2943.short.

223 Institute of Medicine, *Dietary Reference Intakes*, 54–55, 59.

224 A. P. Simopoulos, "The Importance of the Ratio of Omega-6/Omega-3 Essential Fatty Acids," Center for Genetics, Nutrition and Health, Biomedicine, and Pharmacotherapy, 2002), http://www.ncbi.nlm.nih.gov/pubmed/12442909.

sive amounts of omega-6 fatty acids and are deficient in omega-3 fatty acids, with an unbalanced ratio of approximately 16:1. This unhealthy ratio promotes the pathogenesis of many diseases, including cardiovascular disease, cancer, and inflammatory and autoimmune diseases.

Therefore, it is recommended to lower our intake of omega-6 by limiting foods such as soybeans; sunflower, corn, soybean, and cottonseed oils; and foods prepared with these oils. Rather, use canola and olive oils, and increase intake of omega-3 via ground flaxseed and flaxseed oil, chia seed, fish or fish oils, and nuts. Certain vegetables and beans are also high in omega-3.

There are three main types of omega-3 fatty acids:

1. EPA—eicosapentaenoic acid
2. DHA—docosahexaenoic acid. EPA and DHA are both long-chain omega-3 fatty acids, plentiful in fish; algae often provides only DHA
3. ALA—alpha-linolenic acid, a short-chain omega-3 fatty acid, found in plants such as flaxseed

Though beneficial, ALA omega-3 fatty acids have less potent health benefits than EPA and DHA.

Omega-3s are anti-inflammatory, and that could partially explain why many studies suggest that they provide benefits minimizing the risk of a wide range of diseases such as cancer, asthma, depression, cardiovascular disease, ADHD, dementia, and autoimmune diseases like rheumatoid arthritis.

For these and other reasons, the Department of Health and Human Services (HHS), the US Department of Agriculture (USDA), the American Heart Association, and the American Dietetic Association **recommend eating two eight-ounce servings of fish each week.**

Detrimental Fats
Detrimental fats include trans fats, cholesterol, and saturated fats.

Trans fats. In November 2013, the FDA made a preliminary determination that trans fats (partially hydrogenated oils) are no longer generally recognized as safe (GRAS) in human food.

Trans fats (partially hydrolyzed polyunsaturated fats) provide no known benefits to human health. Studies unequivocally demonstrate that the higher the intake of trans fats, the higher the risk of chronic heart disease.

Only very small amounts of trans fats are found in meat and milk products. The vast majority of trans fats ingested by most people are processed, not natural fats.

Trans fats became popular to manufacture because they are cheap, they make food tasty, and they substantially increase the shelf life of the foods they are combined with.

Trans fats increase risk of chronic heart disease via raising the body's bad cholesterol, LDL, and lowering the body's good cholesterol, HDL.

Natural and artificial trans fats are chemically different. Two Canadian studies[225,226] show that the natural trans fat—vaccenic acid—found in beef and dairy products, could actually be beneficial (compared to artificial hydrogenated vegetable shortening) by lowering LDL (the "bad" cholesterol) and triglyceride levels. These studies, however, are disputed. A study by the US Department of Agriculture shows that vaccenic acid raises both HDL (the "good" fat) and LDL cholesterol, whereas industrial trans fats only raise LDL without any beneficial effect on HDL.

Though most authorities don't distinguish between natural and artificial trans fats and recommend limiting the intake of both, there is no disagreement that natural trans fats are found only in *tiny* quantities in foods that are predominantly nutritious, such as beef and dairy. As such, they are of almost no concern in comparison to artificial trans fats, which are consumed in high quantities in the typical Western diet.

225 Red Orbit Staff and Wire Reports, "Trans Fats from Ruminant Animals May Be Beneficial," Red Orbit (September 8, 2011), http://www.redorbit.com/news/health/2608879/trans-fats-from-ruminant-animals-may-be-beneficial/.
226 Chantal M. C. Bassett et al., "Dietary Vaccenic Acid Has Antiatherogenic Effects in LDLr-/- Mice," *Journal of Nutrition* (2010), http://jn.nutrition.org/content/140/1/18.

Artificial trans fats are created in an industrial process that adds hydrogen to liquid vegetable oils to make them more solid.

The American Heart Association puts forth the following recommendations in terms of people limiting their daily intake of trans fats:

1. Read the nutrition facts panel on foods you buy. The primary dietary source for trans fats in processed food is partially hydrogenated oils. However, products can be listed as "zero grams of trans fats" as long as they contain less than 0.5 grams of trans fat per serving. When eating out, ask what kind of oil foods are cooked in. Replace the trans fats in your diet with monounsaturated or polyunsaturated fats.
2. Eat a diet emphasizing fruits, vegetables, whole grains, low-fat dairy products, poultry, fish, and nuts, and limit the amount of red meat and sugary foods and beverages you consume.
3. Primarily use naturally occurring, unhydrogenated vegetable oils such as canola, safflower, sunflower, or olive oil.
4. Look for processed foods made with unhydrogenated oil rather than partially hydrogenated or hydrogenated vegetable oils or saturated fat.
5. Choose soft margarines (liquid or tub varieties) over harder stick forms. Look for "zero grams trans fat" on the nutrition facts label and be sure there are no hydrogenated oils in the ingredients list.
6. Limit commercially baked foods that may contain trans fat such as doughnuts, frozen pizza, cookies, crackers, muffins, and pies and cakes.
7. Limit commercially fried foods made with shortening or partially hydrogenated vegetable oils. These foods are very high in fat and are likely to contain trans fat.

Cholesterol. Intake of high quantities of dietary cholesterol raises LDL for individuals who are hypersensitive to dietary cholesterol (common among diabetics); high LDL levels pose a risk of heart disease. Foods highest in cholesterol are egg yolks, animal organs, butter, whipped cream, cream cheese, and other fatty cheeses. Foods with moderate levels of cholesterol are meat, poultry, fish, and other dairy products. Foods with little cholesterol are cottage cheese, yogurt, and skim milk. Foods with no cholesterol are egg whites, fruits, grains, and nuts.

The United States Department of Health and Human Services used to recommend limiting dietary intake of cholesterol to no more than three hundred milligrams per day. However, in the recent "2015 Scientific Report" of the Dietary Guidelines Advisory Committee, the committee nullified that recommendation, writing, "Available evidence shows no appreciable relationship between consumption of dietary cholesterol and serum (blood) cholesterol." The report concluded that "cholesterol is not a nutrient of concern for overconsumption."[227]

The NLA (National Lipids Association) agrees with the US Department of Health and Human Services only partially, writing, "Observational data have consistently reported no association between dietary cholesterol or egg consumption (a large contributor to dietary cholesterol intake) and ASCVD (arteriosclerotic cardiovascular disease) risk in the general population, but suggest that there may be increased ASCVD risk associated with greater cholesterol and egg consumption in those with diabetes mellitus."[228]

However, the NLA points out that unlike observational data that reports no correlation between dietary cholesterol and cholesterol blood levels, in controlled feeding randomized controlled trials, each one hundred milligrams per day of dietary cholesterol raises LDL-C by an average of 1.9 mg/dL.

---

227   Dietary Guidelines Advisory Committee, "Scientific Report of the Dietary Guidelines," Department of Health and Human Services and Department of Agriculture, (February 2015), http://health.gov/dietaryguidelines/2015-scientific-report/pdfs/scientific-report-of-the-2015-dietary-guidelines-advisory-committee.pdf.

228   National Lipids Association, http://www.lipidjournal.com/pb/assets/raw/Health%20Advance/journals/jacl/NLA_Recommendations_manuscript.pdf.

Therefore, based on the controlled trials, the NLA's (National Lipid Association) recommendations are to limit cholesterol intake to less than two hundred milligrams per day to lower LDL cholesterol. And for known or suspected hyper-responders, further reduction in dietary cholesterol beyond the less than two hundred milligrams per day may be considered. Consumption of very low intakes of dietary cholesterol (near zero mg/day) may be helpful for such individuals.

Saturated fats. Foods high in saturated fats are palm oil, palm kernel oil, and high-fat dairy and meat products. Coconut oil is also high in saturated fats; however, it does not contain the typical long-chain triglyceride saturated fats found in meat and dairy but rather has the medium-chain triglycerides (MCTs). Later it is explained why coconut oil is a uniquely beneficial saturated fat.

Consumption of saturated fats raises LDL cholesterol levels more than the consumption of unsaturated fats.[229] LDL cholesterols clog up arteries, and increased levels of LDL cholesterol are associated with increased risk of cardiovascular disease. Therefore, until recently, it was universally assumed that increased saturated fats would increase the risk of cardiovascular disease.

A new meta-analysis in the Annals of Internal Medicine (2014), which looks at seventy-two published studies involving 530,525 participants, challenges the assumption that increased consumption of saturated fats increases the risk cardiovascular disease.[230, 231] One the-

---

229   R. J. Nicolosi, "Dietary Fat Saturation Effects on Low-Density-Lipoprotein Concentrations and Metabolism in Various Animal Models," *American Journal of Clinical Nutrition* 65, no. 5 (1997), http://ajcn.nutrition.org/content/65/5/1617S.abstract.

230   Rajiv Chowdhury et al., "Association of Dietary, Circulating, and Supplement Fatty Acids with Coronary Risk: A Systematic Review and Meta-Analysis," *Annals of Internal Medicine* 160, no. 6 (March 18, 2014), http://annals.org/article.aspx?articleid=1846638. "Conclusion: Current evidence does not clearly support cardiovascular guidelines that encourage high consumption of polyunsaturated fatty acids and low consumption of total saturated fats."

231   Bazian, "Saturated Fats and Heart Disease Link 'Unproven,'" *Behind the Headlines: Health News from NHS Choices* (March 18, 2014), http://www.nhs.uk/news/2014/03march/pages/saturated-fats-and-heart-disease-link-unproven.aspx.

ory is that the specific types of LDLs raised by increased consumption of saturated fats have no substantial effect on cardiovascular disease. However, the conclusions of this study are disputed,[232] and medical and governmental authorities[233] still maintain the position that saturated fat is a risk factor for cardiovascular disease.

Unlike trans fats, which are nearly nonexistent in animal tissue, saturated fats constitute over a third of total fatty acids in animal tissue.[234] Additionally, trans fats have no benefits to human health, whereas saturated fats do.[235, 236, 237] Finally, even the medical and governmental authorities who are still following the old-school assumptions that consumption of saturated fats is linked to cardiovascular disease do not require completely avoiding consumption of saturated fats. Rather, they allow 7 to 10 percent of total caloric intake from saturated fats. So as long as one isn't gulping down palm oil, it's completely safe to eat products that contain palm and coconut oils. Just avoid consuming large quantities of palm and coconut oil and limit fatty dairy and meat products.

---

232 Walter Willett, Frank Sacks, and Meir Stampfer, "Dietary Fat and Heart Disease Study Is Seriously Misleading," *Nutrition Source*, Harvard School of Public Health (March 19, 2014), http://www.hsph.harvard.edu/nutritionsource/2014/03/19/dietary-fat-and-heart-disease-study-is-seriously-misleading/.

233 World Health Organization, the American Dietetic Association, the Dietitians of Canada, the British Dietetic Association, American Heart Association, the British Heart Foundation, the World Heart Federation, the British National Health Service, the US Food and Drug Administration, and the European Food Safety Authority.

234 Palmitic and stearic acid constitute nearly all the saturated fats in animal tissue, while myristic and lauric acid constitute merely a tiny fraction of the saturated fats.

235 Palmitic acid is involved in the regulation of hormones. And palmitic and myristic acids are involved in cell messaging and immune function.

236 V. Rioux and P. Legrand, "Saturated Fatty Acids: Simple Molecular Structures with Complex Cellular Functions," *Current Opinion in Clinical Nutrition and Metabolic Care* (2007).

237 Philippe Legrand and Vincent Rioux, "The Complex and Important Cellular and Metabolic Functions of Saturated Fatty Acids," *Lipids* (July 13, 2010), http://www.ncbi.nlm.nih.gov/pmc/articles/PMC2974191/.

UNDERSTANDING BLOOD TEST CHOLESTEROL LEVELS: HDL, LDL, AND TRIGLYCERIDE LEVELS

Cholesterol can't dissolve in the blood. It must be transported through the bloodstream by carriers called lipoproteins (lipids encased in proteins). The two types of lipoproteins that carry cholesterol to and from cells are low-density lipoproteins—LDLs—and high-density lipoproteins—HDLs.

LDL cholesterol is considered the "bad" cholesterol because it contributes to plaque, a thick, hard deposit that can clog arteries and make them less flexible. This condition is known as atherosclerosis. If a clot forms and blocks a narrowed artery, a heart attack or stroke can result. Another condition called peripheral artery disease can develop when plaque buildup narrows an artery that supplies blood to the legs.

HDL cholesterol is considered "good" cholesterol because, according to accepted theory, it helps remove LDL cholesterol from the arteries, carrying it to the liver, where it is broken down and passed out of the body. High levels of HDL are beneficial, whereas low levels of HDL cholesterol are associated with increased risk of heart disease.

Triglycerides are used to store excess energy from the diet. High levels of triglycerides in the blood are associated with atherosclerosis and fatty liver disease. Elevated triglycerides can be caused by obesity, physical inactivity, cigarette smoking, excess alcohol consumption, and a diet high in carbohydrates (more than 60 percent of total calories). Underlying diseases or genetic disorders are sometimes the cause of high triglycerides. People with high triglycerides often have a high LDL cholesterol (bad) level and a low HDL cholesterol (good) level. Many people with heart disease or diabetes also have high triglyceride levels.

Blood tests normally show four primary health indicators of different types of lipid levels:

1. **Total cholesterol**
   Desired: ≤ 200 mg/dL
   Borderline high: 200–239 mg/dL
   High: ≥ 240 mg/dL
2. **Triglycerides**
   Normal: ≤ 150 mg/dL
   Borderline high: 150–199 mg/dL
   High: 200–499 mg/dL
   Very high: ≥ 500 mg/dL
3. **HDL cholesterol**
   Low: ≤ 39 mg/dL
   Normal: 40–59 mg/dL
   Desirable: ≥ 60 mg/dL
4. **LDL cholesterol**
   Optimal: ≤ 100 mg/dL
   Near optimal: 100–129 mg/dL
   Borderline high: 130–159 mg/dL
   High: ≥ 160 mg/dL

Total cholesterol includes both HDL and LDL and therefore is a poor indicator of cardiovascular health. It should be ignored when the details of the other three indicators are available. Total cholesterol level can rise due to increased HDL, which is actually beneficial.

The most important of the four indicators are the LDL levels, which are directly responsible for increasing arterial plaque. It is theorized that triglycerides and HDL affect LDL levels and thereby affect arterial plaque, but no conclusive connection has yet been proven as to triglycerides and HDL *causing* heart disease,[238] even though it has been proven that they are indicative of heart disease. Similarly, when lipid levels are indicative of heart condition, reducing LDL levels has been

---

238 R. P. Mensink and M. B. Katan, "Effect of Dietary Fatty Acids on Serum Lipids and Lipoproteins: A Meta-Analysis of 27 Trials," *Arteriosclerosis and Thrombosis: A Journal of Vascular Biology*, American Heart Association (August 1992), http://atvb.ahajournals.org/content/12/8/911.full.pdf?origin=publication_detail.

proven to reduce risk of a heart condition, whereas reducing triglycerides and raising HDL alone (without reducing LDL) may not reduce the risk of a heart disease.

HOW TO REDUCE LDL LEVELS
There are several methods of reducing LDL levels.

Medication
Most doctors will simply prescribe medications (usually statins) that reduce LDL levels if they are too high. Although statins have been shown to reduce the risk of mortality among individuals with clinical history of cardiovascular disease, according to a meta-analysis of eleven randomized controlled trials involving 65,229 participants, statin therapy has not been shown to reduce mortality among intermediate- to high-risk individuals without a history of cardiovascular disease (CVD).[239] Additionally, it is clear that statins carry with them many known and unknown side effects harming health (e.g., diabetes[240] and muscle deterioration[241]). Using them should only be considered as a last resort.

Diet
Excessive calories, carbohydrates, obesity, and high blood sugar levels all contribute to higher LDL levels. Reducing dietary cholesterol[242]

239 K. K. Ray et al., "Statins and All-Cause Mortality in High-Risk Primary Prevention: A Meta-Analysis of 11 Randomized Controlled Trials Involving 65,229 Participants," *Archives of Internal Medicine* (June 28, 2010), http://www.ncbi.nlm.nih.gov/pubmed/20585067.
240 R. Sukhija et al., "Effect of Statins on Fasting Plasma Glucose in Diabetic and Nondiabetic Patients," *Journal of Investigative Medicine* (March 2009), http://www.ncbi.nlm.nih.gov/pubmed/19188844?dopt=Abstract.
241 Stephanie L. Di Stasi et al., "Effects of Statins on Skeletal Muscle: A Perspective for Physical Therapists," *Journal of American Physical Therapy Association* (October 2010), http://www.ncbi.nlm.nih.gov/pmc/articles/PMC2949584/.
242 C. J. Packard et al., "Cholesterol Feeding Increases Low Density Lipoprotein Synthesis," *Journal of Clinical Investigation* (July 1983), http://www.ncbi.nlm.nih.gov/pmc/articles/PMC1129159/.

(found in egg yolks, animal fats and organs, and certain dairy products) helps some individuals (particularly diabetics) reduce their LDL levels.[243]

The National Lipid Association also recommends a high fiber diet and including plant sterols and stanols in your diet. Plant sterols and stanols are substances that occur naturally in small amounts in many grains, vegetables, fruits, legumes, nuts, and seeds. Since they have powerful cholesterol-lowering properties, manufacturers have started adding them to foods. You can now get stanols or sterols in margarine spreads, orange juice, cereals, and even granola bars.

Consumption of trans fats and saturated fats raises LDL levels.[244] However, as previously noted, a new meta-analysis[245] in the *Annals of Internal Medicine* (2014) challenges the assumption that increased consumption of saturated fats increases the risk cardiovascular disease.[246] Palm oil, palm kernel oil, coconut oil, and high-fat dairy and meat products are high in saturated fats and therefore shouldn't be eaten in excess.

Coconut oil, however, is an unusual and beneficial saturated fat. Although high in saturated fats, it does not contain the typical long-chain triglyceride saturated fats found in meat and dairy but rather contains medium-chain triglycerides. Numerous studies show that a relatively low to moderate intake (fifteen to thirty grams per day) of

---

243 National Lipids Association, http://www.lipidjournal.com/pb/assets/raw/Health%20 Advance/journals/jacl/NLA_Recommendations_manuscript.pdf.

244 R. J. Nicolosi, "Dietary Fat Saturation Effects on Low-Density-Lipoprotein Concentrations and Metabolism in Various Animal Models," *American Journal of Clinical Nutrition* 65, no. 5 (1997), http://ajcn.nutrition.org/content/65/5/1617S.abstract.

245 Rajiv Chowdhury et al., "Association of Dietary, Circulating, and Supplement Fatty Acids With Coronary Risk: A Systematic Review and Meta-analysis," *Annals of Internal Medicine*, (March 18, 2014), 160, No. 6." "Conclusion: Current evidence does not clearly support cardiovascular guidelines that encourage high consumption of polyunsaturated fatty acids and low consumption of total saturated fats." http://annals.org/article. aspx?articleid=1846638

246 Bazian, "Saturated Fats and Heart Disease link 'unproven'," *Behind the Headlines*, Health News from NHS Choices, (March 18, 2014).
http://www.nhs.uk/news/2014/03march/pages/saturated-fats-and-heart-disease-link-un-proven.aspx

medium-chain triglycerides, as opposed to long-chain triglycerides, as part of daily diet *enhances daily energy expenditure*[247, 248, 249] and *reduces appetite.*[250, 251] A study of forty obese women who were supplementing with one ounce of coconut oil per day led to a significant reduction in both BMI and waist circumference in a period of twelve weeks.[252] And a study of twenty obese males supplementing with one ounce of coconut oil per day led to a one-inch reduction of waist circumference after just four weeks.[253]

Additionally, 50 percent of the fatty acid in coconut oil is lauric acid, the saturated fatty acid that is most inhibitory against bacteria.[254] It is also considered a medicinal food, as it is very effective in killing the

247   T. B. Seaton et al., "Thermic Effect of Medium-Chain and Long-Chain Triglycerides in Man," *American Journal of Clinical Nutrition* (November 1986), http://www.ncbi.nlm.nih.gov/pubmed/3532757.

248   L Scalfi, A. Coltorti, and F. Contaldo, "Postprandial Thermogenesis in Lean and Obese Subjects after Meals Supplemented with Medium-Chain and Long-Chain Triglycerides," *American Journal of Clinical Nutrition* (May 1991), http://www.ncbi.nlm.nih.gov/pubmed/2021124.

249   A. G. Dulloo et al., "Twenty-Four-Hour Energy Expenditure and Urinary Catecholamines of Humans Consuming Low-to-Moderate Amounts of Medium-Chain Triglycerides: A Dose-Response Study in a Human Respiratory Chamber," *European Journal of Clinical Nutrition* (March 1996), http://www.ncbi.nlm.nih.gov/pubmed/8654328.

250   R. J. Rtubbs and C. G. Harbron, "Covert Manipulation of the Ratio of Medium- to Long-Chain Triglycerides in Isoenergetically Dense Diets: Effect on Food Intake in Ad Libitum Feeding Men," *International Journal of Obesity and Related Metabolic Disorders* (May 1996), http://www.ncbi.nlm.nih.gov/pubmed/8696422.

251   V. van Wymelbeke et al., "Influence of Medium-Chain and Long-Chain Triacylglycerols on the Control of Food Intake in Men," *American Journal of Clinical Nutrition* (August 1998), http://www.ncbi.nlm.nih.gov/pubmed/9701177.

252   M. L. Assunção et al., "Effects of Dietary Coconut Oil on the Biochemical and Anthropometric Profiles of Women Presenting Abdominal Obesity," *Lipids* (July 2009), http://www.ncbi.nlm.nih.gov/pubmed/19437058.

253   Kai Ming Liau et al., "An Open-Label Pilot Study to Assess the Efficacy and Safety of Virgin Coconut Oil in Reducing Visceral Adiposity," *ISRN Pharmacology* (2011), http://www.ncbi.nlm.nih.gov/pmc/articles/PMC3226242/.

254   Jon J. Kabara et al., "Fatty Acids and Derivatives as Antimicrobial Agents," *Antimicrobial Agents and Chemotherapy* (July 1972), http://www.ncbi.nlm.nih.gov/pmc/articles/PMC444260/.

fungus candida,[255] a common source of yeast infections. Nevertheless, the National Lipid Association still recommends keeping saturated fats under 7 percent of total energy intake, even if those saturated fats come from coconut oil.

Reducing total caloric intake, dietary cholesterol, trans[256] and saturated fats, and carbohydrates and maintaining stable blood sugar levels will often reduce LDL levels sufficiently. Studies demonstrate that increasing dietary fiber and consuming green tea[257] and coenzyme Q-10[258] also lowers LDL levels.

For decades, conventional wisdom assumed that dietary fats increase cholesterol levels and risk of heart disease, and it was therefore recommended to replace dietary fats with carbohydrates. However, numerous studies reveal that in general the reverse is true: increasing carbohydrates in place of fats raises serum cholesterol and increases risk of heart disease. A meta-analysis of twenty-seven studies concludes that the "replacement of carbohydrates with fat reduces the fasting level of triglycerides and thus presumably also reduces the level of very-low-density lipoproteins (VLDLs) and other triglyceride-rich particles. More specifically, very-long-chain omega 3 lipids, as found in fish oils, markedly lower serum triglycerides. Replacing carbohydrates with fats also increases HDL; saturated fats increase the HDL more than polyunsaturated fats. However, since saturated fats increase LDL, and

255   D. O. Ogbolu et al., "In Vitro Antimicrobial Properties of Coconut Oil on Candida Species in Ibadan, Nigeria," *Journal of Medicinal Food* (June 2007), http://www.ncbi.nlm.nih.gov/pubmed/17651080.

256   R. P. Mensink and M. B. Katan, "Effect of Dietary Trans Fatty Acids on High-Density and Low-Density Lipoprotein Cholesterol Levels in Healthy Subjects," *New England Journal of Medicine* (August 1990), http://www.ncbi.nlm.nih.gov/pubmed/2374566.

257   X. X. Zheng et al., "Green Tea Intake Lowers Fasting Serum Total and LDL Cholesterol in Adults: A Meta-Analysis of 14 Randomized Controlled Trials," *American Journal of Clinical Nutrition* (August 2011), http://www.ncbi.nlm.nih.gov/pubmed/21715508.

258   H. Ahmadvand et al., "Effects of Coenzyme Q(10) on LDL Oxidation in Vitro," Acta medica Iranica (2013), http://www.ncbi.nlm.nih.gov/pubmed/23456579.

polyunsaturated fats lower LDL, therefore unsaturated fatty acids produce a more favorable lipoprotein profile than saturated fats."[259]

For more studies demonstrating that replacing carbohydrates with
fat reduces the risk of heart disease and for more details concerning
how and why this works, see chapter 14.

Exercise

There are a variety of theories as to *how* exercise reduces LDL levels,
but it is undisputed that exercise is beneficial in this respect—particularly aerobic exercise, according to the National Lipid Association.

Thyroid

Poor thyroid function can contribute to elevated LDL levels.[260, 261]
Certain herbs can support thyroid function, including sage, ashwagand-
ha, *Bacopa monnieri*, and *Coleus forskohlii*. Sufficient iodine and selenium
are also essential for optimal thyroid function.

---

259   Mensink and Katan, "Effect of Dietary Fatty Acids on Serum Lipids and Lipoproteins:
A Meta-Analysis of 27 Trials," *Arteriosclerosis and Thrombosis: A Journal of Vascular Biology*,
American Heart Association (August 1992), http://atvb.ahajournals.org/content/12/8/911.
full.pdf?origin=publication_detail.
260   Evagelos N. Liberopoulos and Moses S. Elisaf, "Dyslipidemia in Patients with
Thyroid Disorders," *Hormones*, Greek Endocrine Society (2002), http://www.hormones.
gr/31/article/article.html.
261   L. H. Duntas, "Thyroid Disease and Lipids," *Thyroid* (April 12, 2002), http://www.
ncbi.nlm.nih.gov/pubmed/12034052. "Hypothyroidism (underactive thyroid) is characterized by hypercholesterolaemia (too much cholesterol) and a marked increase in low-
density lipoproteins (LDL) and apolipoprotein B (apo A) because of a decreased fractional
clearance of LDL by a reduced number of LDL receptors in the liver. Cardiac oxygen
consumption is reduced in hypothyroidism. Hypothyroidism is often accompanied by
diastolic hypertension that, in conjunction with the dyslipidemia, may promote atherosclerosis. Thyroxine therapy, in a thyrotropin (TSH)-suppressive dose, usually leads to a
considerable improvement of the lipid profile. The changes in lipoproteins are correlated
with changes in free thyroxine (FT(4)) levels. Subclinical (mild) hypothyroidism (SH) is
associated with lipid disorders that are characterized by normal or slightly elevated total
cholesterol levels, increased LDL, and lower HDL. Moreover, SH has been associated with
endothelium dysfunction, aortic atherosclerosis, and myocardial infarction. Lipid disorders
exhibit great individual variability. Nevertheless, they might be a link, although it has not
been proved, between SH and atherosclerosis."

If thyroid function is severely impaired, thyroid hormone replacement may be warranted.

Bacteria

Studies have demonstrated that there is a correlation between the *Helicobacter pylori* infection and elevated LDL cholesterol levels.[262] The cause and effect are yet unclear. Two other bacteria, *Chlamydia pneumonia* and cytomegalovirus, are also implicated in raising LDL levels.[263]

If one is infected with *Helicobacter pylori*, medical treatment removing the bacteria could significantly reduce LDL levels.

Sucralose

Sucralose is an artificial noncaloric sweetener commonly used to sweeten "health" foods and "diet" foods. Aside from numerous other harmful side effects, studies have demonstrated that sucralose raises LDL levels.[264] For those who regularly consume sucralose, avoiding it could lower LDL levels.

---

262 Hack-Lyoung Kim et al., "Helicobacter Pylori Infection is Associated with Elevated Low Density Lipoprotein Cholesterol Levels in Elderly Koreans," *Journal of Korean Med Science* (May 2011), http://www.ncbi.nlm.nih.gov/pmc/articles/PMC3082118/.

263 A. Al-Ghamdi, A. A. Jiman-Fatani, and H. El-Banna, "Role of Chlamydia Pneumoniae, Helicobacter Pylori and Cytomegalovirus in Coronary Artery Disease," *Pakistan Journal of Pharmaceutical Sciences* (April 24, 2011), http://www.ncbi.nlm.nih.gov/pubmed/21454155.

264 Helen N. Saada et al., "Biological Effect of Sucralose in Diabetic Rats," *Food and Nutrition Sciences* 4, no.7A (July 2013), http://www.scirp.org/journal/PaperInformation. aspx?PaperID=34006.

Appendix to Chapter 13

Understanding the Terms Saturated, Unsaturated, Polyunsaturated, Cis, and Trans

Ninety-eight percent of dietary fats are triacylglycerol—a glycerol molecule esterified with three fatty acid molecules.[265] The fatty acids molecules vary in type. They can be either saturated or unsaturated.

---

265 It is also esterified with smaller amounts of phospholipids and sterols.

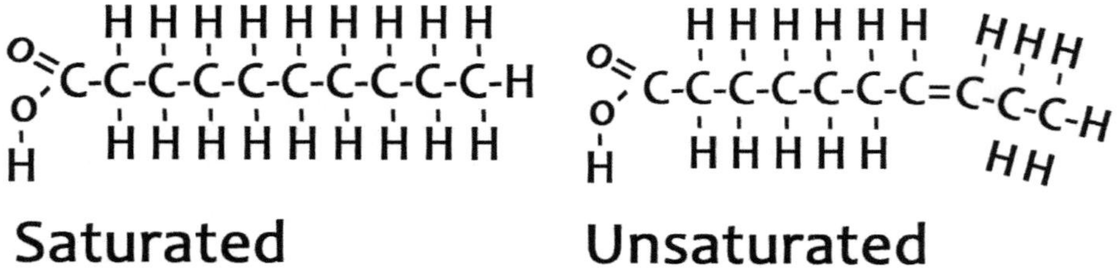

$$O=C_O^{-}-C-C-C-C-C-C-C-C-C-H$$

Saturated

Unsaturated

Figure A13-1. The respective structures of saturated and unsaturated fatty acids

To understand the chemical difference, it is useful to visualize them (figure A13-1). Fatty acids are primarily a chain of carbon molecules. Each carbon molecule has four bonds. In saturated fatty acids, the carbon molecules in the chain use one bond to connect to the carbon before it and another bond to connect to the next carbon in the chain. The other two remaining bonds are "saturated" by being individually connected to two separate hydrogen molecules. In unsaturated fatty acids, at least one of those carbon molecules has an "unsaturated" bond, meaning it only uses one bond to be connected to one hydrogen molecule, enabling its fourth bond to make a second (double) bond with one of the carbons that it is connected to. Were that double bond to become a single bond and use the freed-up bond to connect to a hydrogen molecule, it would become saturated.

In review, saturated fatty acids are carbon chains without double bonds, and unsaturated fatty acids are carbon chains connected by double bonds (which can be saturated by adding hydrogen atoms to them, converting the double bonds to single bonds).

Unsaturated fatty acids are further divided into the following categories:

- **Trans**: these are harmful (*trans* is Latin for "opposite").
- **Cis**: these are beneficial (*cis* is Latin for "side by side").

As shown in figure A13-2 (top), in a *cis* configuration, adjacent hydrogen atoms are on the same side of the double bond, whereas in the *trans* configuration, the adjacent hydrogen atoms are opposite each other.

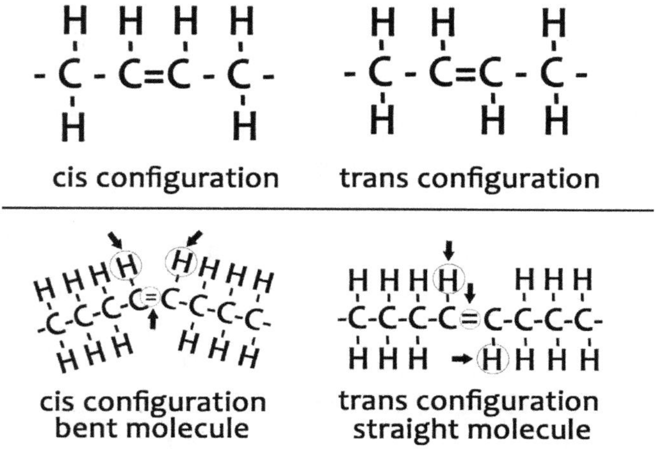

Figure A13-2. The respective structures of *cis* and *trans* unsaturated fatty acids.

Top left—adjacent hydrogen atoms on same side.
Top right—adjacent hydrogen atoms on opposite sides.
Bottom—the bending effect in cis configuration.

As shown in figure A13-2 (bottom), in cis configuration, the two adjacent hydrogen atoms cause the carbon chain to bend. When a chain has many cis bonds, it becomes quite curved (figure A13-3).

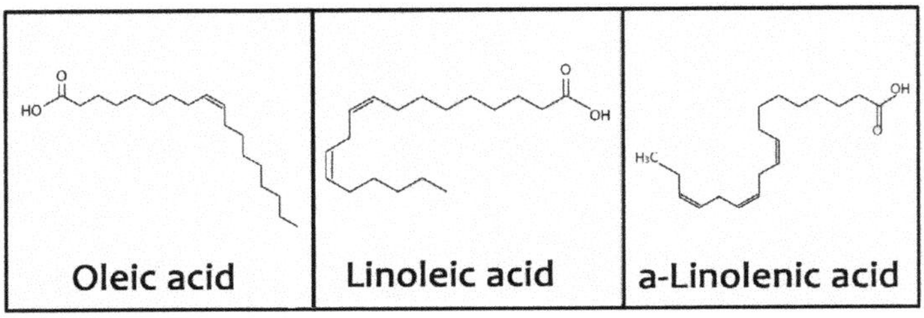

| Oleic acid | Linoleic acid | a-Linolenic acid |

Figure A13-3. An illustration of the bending effects of three different cis unsaturated acids: *oleic acid*—one double bond, *linoleic acid*—two double bonds, and *alpha-linolenic acid*—three double bonds.

For example, oleic acid, with one double bond, has a "kink" in it, whereas linoleic acid, with two double bonds, has a more pronounced bend. Alpha-linolenic acid, with three double bonds, is hook shaped (figure A10-3). The effect of this is that the cis bonds limit the ability of fatty acids to be closely packed and therefore usually cause them to melt into a liquid at a lower temperature, whereas in the trans configuration, the nearly identical fatty acid remains tightly packed, solid (not melted), doesn't need refrigeration, and has longer shelf life.

Unsaturated fatty acids (both trans and cis) are further divided into:

- Monounsaturated—only one double bond
- Polyunsaturated—more than one double bond

Polyunsaturated fats are further divided into:

- Omega-3—includes three types fatty acids involved in human physiology: EPA (eicosapentaenoic acid) and DHA (docosahexaenoic acid), which are commonly found in marine oils, and ALA (alpha-linolenic acid), found in plant oils.
- Omega-6 (linoleic acid)
- Omega-9 (oleic acid)
- Conjugated fatty acids
- Other polyunsaturated fatty acids

Part IV

Comparative Study of Popular Diets

An Examination of Many Studies Determining the Most Effective Methods for Weight Loss and Improvement of Metabolic Parameters

14

Benefits of Low-Carbohydrate Diets

The fourth primary element for alleviating the metabolic syndrome is measured glycemic load. For most people, a measured glycemic load includes a *reduction* in carbohydrates and limiting high-GI carbohydrates. Chapter 10 explained that the RDA of carbohydrates of 45 to 65 percent is too high, according to many experts. This is especially true for people with the metabolic syndrome—obesity, high blood sugar, high serum cholesterol, and/or high blood pressure.

This chapter individually summarizes twenty-one studies that concluded that lower the percentage of carbohydrates, the more effective the diets are in reducing body fat and stabilizing blood sugar. I specifically included studies that dramatically demonstrated the benefits of low-carbohydrate diets. There are other studies whose conclusions are not so dramatic. But I challenge the reader to find even a single study that comes to the opposite conclusion—that high-carbohydrate diets are more effective in reducing body fat and stabilizing blood sugar. I conclude this chapter with six meta-analyses—studies that examine all low-carbohydrate studies—to get a broad and objective picture.

This chapter begins with one particular three-month study published in the journal *Lipids* in 2009. This study is outstanding in regard to the wide array of physiological measurements that were tracked and the efforts made in making the results as accurate as possible. It also has outstanding instructional value as well.

Examples of the researchers' efforts to make the study as precise as possible include the following:

1. They excluded candidates using glucose-lowering, lipid-lowering, or vasoactive prescriptions or supplements; those who had recently been on a carbohydrate-restricted diet; and those who had lost more than five kilograms in the three months preceding the study.

2. They provided subjects with individual and personalized dietary counseling by registered dietitians prior to the dietary intervention. They also provided them with detailed dietary booklets specific to each dietary treatment outlining dietary goals, lists of appropriate foods, recipes, sample meal plans, and food record log sheets. They additionally gave participants weekly follow-up counseling during which body mass was measured, compliance was assessed, and further dietetic education was provided. Seven-day weighed food records were kept during weeks one, six, and twelve of the intervention; the foods recorded were analyzed for energy and macronutrient or micronutrient content using Nutritionist Pro (a cutting edge nutrient analysis system).

As stated earlier, five conditions are associated with the metabolic syndrome according to the National Heart Lung and Blood Institute of the US Department of Health and Human Services:[266]

1. A large waistline
2. A high-triglyceride level
3. A low HDL-cholesterol level
4. High blood pressure
5. High fasting blood sugar

The study examines the effects of a very low-carbohydrate diet on all of the conditions of the metabolic syndrome. What drove the researchers to examine this was the realization that hyperinsulinemia

---

266 National Heart Lung and Blood Institute of the US Department of Health and Human Services, http://www.nhlbi.nih.gov/health/health-topics/topics/ms/.

worsens all of the above conditions and that the consumption of carbo-hydrates increases the body's production and release of insulin.

Traditionally, medicine has treated each of the previous five condi-tions separately. There is a variety of medications that treat high blood sugar. A different group of medications treat high blood pressure. Other medicines attempt to raise HDL; still others attempt to lower triglyceride and LDL levels. This study, however, proves that merely by following a very low-carbohydrate diet, people can improve all these conditions at the same time and lose weight faster than with a low-fat diet consuming the same amount of calories.

Three-Month Study Published in Lipids (2009):[267]

Forty subjects with atherogenic dyslipidemia (the simultaneous conditions of high LDL cholesterol, high triglycerides, and low HDL) were random-ized to either a low-carbohydrate diet, where the ratio of carbohydrates to fat to protein was 12:59:28, or to a low-fat diet, where the ratio of carbo-hydrates to fat to protein was 56:24:20. The diets were followed for twelve weeks. Although the participants were not specifically counseled to reduce calories, there was a reduction in total caloric intake in both groups. The average intake of participants on the low-carbohydrate diet was 1,504 calo-ries versus 1,478 calories for those on the low-fat diet.

Weight Loss

- *10.1 kilograms versus 5.2 kilograms*

Despite similar reductions in calories, weight loss in the carbohy-drate-restricted diet group was, on average, twofold greater than in the low-fat control group (10.1 kg vs. 5.2 kg). There was substantial indi-vidual variation between participants, but nine of twenty subjects in the carbohydrate-restricted diet group lost 10 percent of their starting

---

267 J. S. Volek et al., "Carbohydrate Restriction Has a More Favorable Impact on the Metabolic Syndrome than a Low Fat Diet," *Lipids* (2009), http://link.springer.com/arti-cle/10.1007/s11745-008-3274-2/fulltext.html.

weight—more than all of the subjects in the low-fat diet group. Indeed, none of the subjects following the low-fat diet lost as much weight as the average amount of weight lost in the experimental group.

Glycemic and Insulin Improvement

- *Fasting glucose: –12 percent versus 0 percent*
- *Fasting insulin: –49 percent versus –17 percent*
- *HOMA insulin resistance measurement: –55 percent versus –18 percent*

The carbohydrate-restricted diet resulted in a significant average reduction in fasting glucose of 12 percent. Responses in the low-fat-diet control group were variable, with little average change. Fasting insulin responses were also decreased to a greater extent for subjects following the carbohydrate-restricted diet than for subjects following the low-fat diet (–49% vs. –17%), as were postprandial insulin responses to a meal high in fat (–49% vs. –6%). Similarly, the homeostasis model assessment (HOMA), a measure of insulin resistance, was reduced a greater extent in subjects following the carbohydrate-restricted diet than for subjects in the control group (–55% vs. –18%).

Retinol-binding protein 4 (RBP4) is an adipokine (cell signaling proteins secreted by adipose tissue) that contributes to insulin resistance. Changes in serum RBP4 levels show a significantly greater reduction in subjects consuming the carbohydrate-restricted diet (from 34.6 on average to 27.6 µg/mL) compared to low-fat diet (from 37.1 on average to 39.0 µg/mL).

Cardiovascular Disease Risk Marker Improvements

- *Fasting triacylglycerol levels: –57 percent versus –24 percent*
- *HDL: +10 percent versus –2 percent*
- *ApoB/ApoA–1 ratio: –16 percent versus +8 percent*
- *Plus a beneficial shift from smaller (LDL-3) to larger (LDL-1)*

The hormonal milieu associated with dietary carbohydrate restriction is proposed to create a unique metabolic state characterized by enhanced reliance on lipid sources, more efficient processing of dietary fat, and reduced lipogenesis (converting excess glucose to fats).

The reductions in triacylglycerols associated with the carbohydrate-restricted diet are particularly striking: triacylglycerols were reduced by 57 percent in response to the carbohydrate-restricted diet, compared to 24 percent in response to the low-fat diet. This effect was probably due to decreased lipogenesis (the process of converting sugars to fatty acids) and VLDL-triacylglycerol secretion in addition to increased VLDL-triacylglycerol clearance. Fasting triacylglycerol levels were reduced by 57 percent in response to the carbohydrate-restricted diet, compared to 24 percent in response to the low-fat diet.

HDL cholesterol levels rose more than 10 percent in the carbohydrate-restricted diet, versus a 2 percent drop in the low-fat diet. Considering the established importance of increasing HDL-C as a therapeutic target for men and women, the effect on HDL-C is an important result from this and other studies.

Apolipoprotein B (ApoB) leads to plaques that cause vascular disease. Considerable evidence shows that levels of ApoB are a better indicator of heart disease risk than total cholesterol or LDL.

The ApoB/Apo A-1 ratio improved in subjects following the carbohydrate-restricted diet but was slightly worse on average for subjects of the low-fat diet (–16% vs. +8%).

LDL particles vary in size and density, and studies show that a pattern that has a greater number of small, dense LDL particles equates to a higher risk factor for coronary heart disease than does a pattern with more of the *larger and less dense* LDL particles.

LDL-particle redistribution in subjects following the carbohydrate-restricted diet reflects a beneficial shift from smaller (LDL-3) to larger (LDL-1) particles, whereas there is little change in the concentration or size of LDL particles on the low-fat diet.

Dietary and Plasma Levels of Saturated Fatty Acid

Old school thought assumed that higher levels of dietary fat consumed would lead to higher levels of fatty acids in the blood plasma. But studies have shown that carbohydrate-restricted diets, although often relatively high in saturated fatty acids, show very beneficial effects on plasma fatty acids compared to those seen in studies of moderate to high dietary carbohydrates. A high-carbohydrate diet prolongs circulatory exposure to dietary saturated fatty acid, and conversely, dietary restriction of carbohydrates reduces secretion of insulin, thereby allowing for greater rates of lipid oxidation and management of the incoming lipid mix. High dietary fat is thus only harmful if there are sufficient carbohydrates to provide the hormonal state in which the fat will be stored rather than oxidized. The carbohydrate-restricted diet with a greater proportion of fat and saturated fat leads to a reduction in plasma-saturated fatty acids, particularly palmitic acid (whose presence has been linked to higher levels of fat storage). The carbohydrate-restricted diet also reduces the amount of excess blood sugar that is converted to fat for storage.

OTHER STUDIES COMPARING LOW-CARBOHYDRATE DIETS TO OTHER DIETS

Whereas the above study was performed meticulously, there are many more studies with similar conclusions comparing low-carbohydrate diets to a control group or to other diets. I have selected the following twenty studies as they support my understanding that low-carbohydrate, high-protein diets are the most beneficial for short-term (up to six months) weight loss and the most beneficial for long-term management of blood sugar levels. In the section following immediately this section, I have included six meta-analyses that compare all relevant studies that meet their inclusion requirements. The advantage of meta-analysis studies is that they don't cherry-pick just the studies that support the authors' theses. Yet despite the objectivity of the meta-analyses, their results also attest to the benefits of the low-carbohydrate diet, although not as dramatically as the studies that

I have selected. The following twenty studies are arranged in order from shortest to longest, ranging in duration between six weeks up to a full year.

Six-Week Study Published in the Journal of the American Dietetic Association (2005)[268]

- *Weight: –5.7 percent versus –3.3 percent*
- *Less hunger*

Twenty-three overweight, premenopausal women, age thirty-two to forty-five years, consumed either a low-carbohydrate, high-protein diet or a high-carbohydrate, low-fat diet for six weeks. The low-carbohydrate, high-protein diet involved eating less than twenty grams of carbohydrates a day for first two weeks, then increasing the amount by five grams per week, to reach forty grams of carbohydrates a day at week six with no caloric restriction. The high-carbohydrate, low-fat diet involved eating 1,500 to 1,700 calories per day (with 60% of calories coming from carbohydrates, 15% from protein, and 25% from fat).

The study concludes: "All women experienced a reduction in body weight, but relative body weight loss was greater in the low-carb/high-protein vs. High-carb/low-fat group at week six (5.7% vs. 3.3%). Additionally, subjects complying with low-carb/high-protein diet reported less hunger."

268 S. M. Nickols-Richardson et al., "Perceived Hunger Is Lower and Weight Loss Is Greater in Overweight Premenopausal Women Consuming a Low-Carbohydrate/High-Protein vs. High-Carbohydrate/Low-Fat Diet," *Journal of the American Dietetic Association* (2005), http://www.nel.gov/worksheet.cfm?worksheet_id=250712.

Seven-Week Study Published in Nutrition
and Metabolism (2004)[269]

- *Weight (men): men –6.4 kilograms (–14.1 lb.) versus –3.7 kilograms (–8.1 lb.)*
- *Weight (women): –2.9 kilograms (–6.4 lb.) versus –1.2 kilograms (–2.6 lb.)*

In a randomized, balanced, "two-diet-period" clinical intervention study, twenty-eight subjects (fifteen men and thirteen women) were prescribed two energy-restricted (–500 cal/day) diets: a very low-carbohydrate diet with a goal of decreasing carbohydrate levels below 10 percent of energy and inducing ketosis, and a low-fat diet with a goal similar to national recommendations (60% carbohydrates; 25% fat; 15% protein).

Men consumed both of the diets alternately for two fifty-day periods, whereas women consumed the diets for approximately thirty days each. Subjects switched to the opposite diet after completion of the first diet period (phase II), after which the same measurements were assessed. This experimental approach allowed a comparison of these two diets in two ways: (a) a *between*-group comparison between group a, in which participants consumed the very low-carbohydrate diet, and group b, in which participants consumed the low-fat diet during phase I; and (b) a *within*-group comparison contrasting how the subjects within each group fared on each of the two diets.

Actual nutrient intakes taken from food records during the very low-carbohydrate diet, where the ratio of carbohydrates to protein to fat was 9:63:28, and the low-fat diet, with a ratio of 58:22:20, were significantly different. Dietary energy was restricted but was higher during the very low-carbohydrate diet (1855 calories per day) compared to the low-fat diet (1562 calories per day) for men.

---

269   J. S. Volek et al., "Comparison of Energy-Restricted Very-Low-Carbohydrate and Low-Fat Diets on Weight Loss and Body Composition in Overweight Men and Women," *Nutrition and Metabolism* (2004), http://www.ncbi.nlm.nih.gov/pmc/articles/PMC538279/#B9.

The study concludes,

Both between and within group comparisons revealed a distinct advantage of a very-low-carb diet over a low-fat diet for weight loss (men 6.4 kg. vs. 3.7 and women 2.9 vs. 1.2), total fat loss, and trunk fat loss for men (despite significantly greater energy intake). The majority of women also responded more favorably to the very-low-carb diet, especially in terms of trunk fat loss. Absolute resting energy expenditure (cal/day) was decreased with both diets as expected, but resting energy expenditure expressed relative to body mass (cal/kg), was better maintained on the very-low-carb diet for men only. Individual responses clearly show the majority of men and women experience greater weight and fat loss on a very-low-carb diet than a low-fat diet.

This study shows a clear benefit of a very-low-carb diet over a low-fat diet for short-term body weight and fat loss, especially in men. A preferential loss of fat in the trunk region with a very-low-carb diet is novel and potentially clinically significant but requires further validation. These data provide additional support for the concept of metabolic advantage with diets representing extremes in macronutrient distribution.

Eight-Week Study Published in Metabolic Syndrome and Related Disorders (2003)[270]

- *Weight: –11.46 pounds versus +5.19 pounds*

Obese children from the pediatric endocrinology clinic were prospectively recruited for the study. Children and their parents were allowed to choose one of two dietary protocols: a carbohydrate-restricted diet (<30 g/day, with unlimited calories, protein, and fat; in other words,

---

270   J. R. Bailes et al., "Effect of Low-Carbohydrate, Unlimited Calorie Diet on the Treatment of Childhood Obesity: A Prospective Controlled Study," *Metabolic Syndrome and Related Disorders* (2003), http://www.ncbi.nlm.nih.gov/pubmed/18370665.

a high-protein, low-carbohydrate diet) or a calorie-restricted diet (low-calorie diet).

After two months, children on the high-protein, low-carbohydrate diet lost an average of 11.46 pounds and decreased their BMI by 2.42, compared to the children in the low-calorie diet, who *gained* an average of 5.19 pounds and 1.00 point on the BMI value.

The study concludes that a high-protein, low-carbohydrate, unlimited-calorie diet is superior to a restricted-calorie protocol for weight loss in obese school-age children; moreover, compliance is better. (Since studies[271] show that high protein diets are more satiating, and more effective in burning fat and reducing calorie intake, I can only assume these are the reasons for better adherence to the high protein diet.)

Eight-Week Study Published in Diabetologia (2005)[272]

- *Weight: People on high-fat and high-protein diets lost six pounds more than those on the high-carbohydrate diet.*

Ninety-six normoglycaemic, insulin-resistant women (BMI above 27) were randomized to one of three dietary interventions: a high-carbohydrate, high-fiber (HC) diet, the high-fat (HF) Atkins diet, or the high-protein (HP) Zone diet. The recommendations involved advice concerning food choices and were not prescriptive in terms of total energy. There were supervised weight-loss and weight-maintenance phases (eight weeks each).

Body weight, waist circumference, triglycerides, and insulin levels decreased with all three diets, but, apart from insulin, the reductions were

---

271   T. L. Halton and F. B. Hu, "The Effects of High Protein Diets on Thermogenesis, Satiety and Weight Loss: A Critical Review," *Journal of the American College of Nutrition* (2004), http://www.colorado.edu/intphys/Class/IPHY3700_Greene/pdfs/discussionEssay/thermogenesisSatiety/HaltonProtein2004.pdf.

272   K. A. McAuley et al., "Comparison of High-Fat and High-Protein Diets with a High-Carbohydrate Diet in Insulin-Resistant Obese Women," *Diabetologia* (2005), http://www.ncbi.nlm.nih.gov/pubmed/15616799.

significantly greater in the HF and HP groups than in the HC group. The popular diets reduced insulin resistance to a greater extent than the standard dietary advice did. When compared with the HC diet, the HF and HP diets were shown to produce significantly greater reductions in several parameters, including weight loss (HF: –2.8 kg; HP: –2.7 kg); waist circumference (HF: –3.5 cm; HP –2.7 cm); and triglycerides (HF: –0.30 mmol/l; HP –0.22 mmol/l). LDL cholesterol decreased in individuals on the HC and HP diets but tended to fluctuate in those on the HF diet, to the extent that overall levels were significantly lower in the HP group than in the HF group. Of those on the HF diet, 25 percent showed a greater than 10 percent increase in LDL cholesterol, whereas this occurred in only 13 percent of subjects on the HC diet and 3 percent of those on the HP diet.

This study concludes that a reduced-carbohydrate, higher-protein diet may be the most appropriate overall approach to reducing the risk of cardiovascular disease and type 2 diabetes. The HF approach appears to be successful for weight loss in the short term, but lipid levels should be monitored. The potential deleterious effects of the diet in the long term remain a concern.

Eight-Week Study Published in the International Journal of Food Sciences and Nutrition (2009)[273]

- *Weight: –8.3 percent versus –5.5 percent*

Nineteen obese middle-aged men were randomized to follow one of the two diets. The first diet was a high-carbohydrate diet where the ratio of carbohydrates to fat to protein was 55:30:15. The second option was a high-protein diet with a ratio of 30:30:40. Both diets were followed over an eight-week period.

The HP diet produced a greater weight loss (–8.3% vs. –5.5%) than the HC diet.

---

273 I. Abete et al., "Effects of Two Energy-Restricted Diets Differing in the Carbohydrate/Protein Ratio on Weight Loss and Oxidative Changes of Obese Men," *International Journal of Food Sciences and Nutrition* (2009), http://www.ncbi.nlm.nih.gov/pubmed/18654910.

Nine-Week Study Published in the American
Journal of Clinical Nutrition (1971)[274]

- *Weight, very low-carbohydrate diet: −16.2 kilograms (Weight loss came more from fat than lean mass in this diet)*
- *Weight, low-carbohydrate diet: −12.8 kilograms*
- *Weight, moderate-carbohydrate diet: −11.9 kilograms*

This study compares the effects of three diets equal in total calories and total protein (115 grams per day) on weight loss and body composition in eight obese men. The diets contained varying carbohydrate contents (30, 60, and 104 grams per day), and all food intake was weighed at a special diet table. After nine weeks, weight loss was 16.2, 12.8, and 11.9 kilograms respectively, and fat accounted for 95 percent, 84 percent, and 75 percent of the weight lost, respectively. This demonstrates clearly that lowering carbohydrates is the most effective way to lose weight in the short term.

Ten-Week Study Published in Forum of Nutrition (2003)[275]

- *Weight: nearly ten pound greater average weight loss on the low-carbohydrate, high-protein diet*

Eleven obese (BMI >30) women were randomized to either a moderate-carbohydrate energy-restricted diet with a carbohydrate to fat to protein ratio of 55:30:15, or low-carbohydrate, high-protein energy-restricted diet with a ratio of 40:30:30. The diets were followed during a ten-week dietary intervention study.

---

274   C. M. Young et al., "Effect of Body Composition and Other Parameters in Obese Young Men of Carbohydrate Level of Reduction Diet," *American Journal of Clinical Nutrition* (1971), http://ajcn.nutrition.org/content/24/3/290.full.pdf+html.

275   I. Labayen et al., "Effects of Protein vs. Carbohydrate-Rich Diets on Fuel Utilisation in Obese Women during Weight Loss," *Forum of Nutrition* (2003), http://www.ncbi.nlm.nih.gov/pubmed/15806847.

On average, the individuals on the HP dietary group lost 9.7 pounds more than those in the HC program, mainly due to a fat-mass loss, with no statistical differences in lean body-mass reduction.

The study concludes that the replacement of some dietary carbohydrates by protein in energy-restricted diets improves weight and fat loss and specifically promotes body fat burning in the fasting state, without significant difference in lean body-mass depletion.

Three-Month Study Published in the Journal of Pediatrics (2003)[276]

- *Weight: –21.8 pounds versus –9.0 pounds*

The Atherosclerosis Prevention Referral Center conducted a randomized, controlled twelve-week trial of thirty subjects. The low-carbohydrate group was instructed to consume less than twenty grams of carbohydrates per day for two weeks followed by less than forty grams a day for ten weeks, and the group was also told to eat low-carbohydrate foods according to hunger. The low-fat group was instructed to consume less than 30 percent of energy from fat. The participants' diet composition and weight were monitored and recorded every two weeks. Their serum lipid profiles were obtained at the start of the study and after twelve weeks.

The low-carbohydrate group lost more weight (21.8 lb. vs. 9.0 lb.) and had improvement in non–HDL cholesterol levels. There was improvement in LDL cholesterol levels in the low-fat group but not in the low-carbohydrate group. There were no adverse effects on the lipid profiles of participants in either group.

The study concludes that the low-carbohydrate diet appears to be an effective method for short-term weight loss in overweight adolescents and does not harm the lipid profile.

---

276 S. B. Sondike, N. Copperman, and M. S. Jacobson, "Effects of A Low-Carbohydrate Diet on Weight Loss and Cardiovascular Risk Factor in Overweight Adolescents," *Journal of Pediatrics* (2003), http://www.ncbi.nlm.nih.gov/pubmed/12640371.

Three-Month Study Published in the Archives of Internal Medicine (2004)[277]

- *Weight: –13.6 pounds versus –7.5 pounds*
- *Plus improved lipid levels*

The Mount Sinai Medical Center of Miami Beach, Florida, the largest independent nonprofit teaching hospital in South Florida, conducted a twelve-week study where sixty overweight individuals were randomized, comparing the US National Cholesterol Education Program (NCEP) diet to a moderately low-carbohydrate diet. The NCEP diet had a carbohydrate to fat to protein ratio of 55:30:15, while the moderately low-carbohydrate diet had a ratio of 28:39:33. The low-carbohydrate diet had a two-week induction phase of only 10 percent carbohydrates. Both diets provided approximately 1,300 calories for women and 1,600 calories for men.

The study concludes, "Weight loss was significantly greater in the low-carb group (13.6 lb) than in the NCEP group (7.5 lb), a difference of 6.1 lb. There were also significantly favorable changes in all lipid levels within the low-carb group but not within the NCEP group."

Three-Month Study Published in Diabetic Medicine (2006)[278]

- *Weight: –7.8 pounds versus –2 pounds*
- *Plus improved lipid levels*

In a study of 102 patients with type 2 diabetes who were random-ized to a low-carbohydrate or a low-fat diet for three months, weight

---

277 Y. Wady Aude et al., "The National Cholesterol Education Program Diet vs. a Diet Lower in Carbohydrates and Higher in Protein and Monounsaturated Fat," *Archives of Internal Medicine* (2004), http://archinte.jamanetwork.com/article.aspx?articleid=217514.

278 M. E. Daly et al., "Short-Term Effects of Severe Dietary Carbohydrate-Restriction Advice in Type 2 Diabetes," *Diabetic Medicine* (2006), http://www.ncbi.nlm.nih.gov/pubmed/16409560.

loss was greater in the low-carbohydrate group (–7.8 lb. vs. –2 lb.), and the HDL cholesterol ratio improved.

Three-Month Study Published in Diabetic Medicine (2007)[279]

- *Weight: –15.2 pounds versus –4.6 pounds*

In a three-month study comparing thirteen diabetic and thirteen nondiabetic individuals randomized to a low-carbohydrate diet, or a "healthy-eating" diet that followed the Diabetes UK recommendations (a calorie restricted, low-fat diet), weight loss was more than triple in the low-carbohydrate group (–15.2 lb. vs. –4.6 lb.) and was equally effective in those with and without diabetes.

Four-Month Study Published in Nutrition and Metabolism (2008)[280]

Comparison of a high-protein diet versus a high-carbohydrate diet

- *Weight: –9.1 percent versus –7.3 percent*
- *Fat loss: –8.7 percent versus –5.7 percent*
- *triacylglycerol: –34 percent versus –14 percent*
- *improved insulin: –34 percent versus –1 percent*

279 P. A. Dyson, S. Beatty, and D. R. Matthew, "A Low-Carbohydrate Diet Is More Effective in Reducing Body Weight than Healthy Eating in Both Diabetic and Non-Diabetic Subjects," *Diabetic Medicine* (2007), http://www.ncbi.nlm.nih.gov/pubmed/17971178.
280 Denise A. Walker Lasker, Ellen M. Evans, and Donald K. Layman, "Moderate Carbohydrate, Moderate Protein Weight Loss Diet Reduces Cardiovascular Disease Risk Compared To High Carbohydrate, Low Protein Diet In Obese Adults: A Randomized Clinical Trial," *Nutrition and Metabolism* (2008). http://www.nutritionandmetabolism.com/content/5/1/30.

Fifty middle-aged obese adults consumed energy-restricted diets (deficit of approximately five hundred cal/day): either high-protein (1.6 g/day of protein per kg of body weight and <170 g/day of carbohydrates) or high-carbohydrate (0.8 g/day of protein per kg of body weight and >220 g/day of carbohydrates) for four months.

The study found that the high-protein dieters lost more weight (–9.1% vs. –7.3%) with a significant reduction in the percent of fat mass compared to high-carbohydrate dieters (–8.7% vs. –5.7%). High-protein dieters also favored reductions in triacylglycerol (–34% vs. –14%) and increases in HDL-C (+5% vs. –3%); however, high-carbohydrate dieters favored reduction in LDL-C (–7% vs. +2.5%). Insulin responses were improved with high-protein dieters compared to high-carbohydrate dieters at both one hour after meals (–34.3% vs. –1.0%) and two hours after meals (–9.2% vs. +46.2%).

The study concludes that a weight-loss diet with moderate-carbohydrate, moderate-protein results in improved changes in body composition, dyslipidemia, and postprandial INS response compared to a high-carbohydrate, low-protein diet. This suggests additional benefits beyond weight management including reduction of metabolic disease.

Six-Month Study Published in the Journal of Clinical Endocrinology and Metabolism (2003)[281]

- *Weight: –18.7 pounds versus –8.6 pounds*

Ironically, a study sponsored by the American Heart Association comparing the effects of a very low-carbohydrate (Atkins) diet to a low-fat diet conforming to the guidelines currently recommended by the

---

281 Bonnie J. Brehm et al., "A Randomized Trial Comparing a Very Low Carbohydrate Diet and a Calorie-Restricted Low Fat Diet on Body Weight and Cardiovascular Risk Factors in Healthy Women," *Journal of Clinical Endocrinology and Metabolism* (2003), http://press.endocrine.org/doi/full/10.1210/jc.2002-021480.

American Heart Association concludes that the very low-carbohydrate (Atkins) diet is more than doubly effective than the American Heart Association's low-fat diet for short-term weight loss. The study also found that even over six months, the Atkins diet is not associated with deleterious effects on important cardiovascular risk factors. The study was performed at the General Clinical Research Center of Cincinnati Children's Hospital Medical Center, where fifty-three healthy obese women were randomized to six months of the comparative diets. The study focused on the relative effects on weight loss and cardiovascular risk factors.

The study concludes, "The women in the low-carb group lost an average of 18.7 lbs, while the low-fat group lost an average of 8.6 lbs. In respect to body fat lost, the low-carb group lost an average of 10.6 lbs, vs. 4.4 lbs in the low-fat group."

Six-Month Study Published in the Annals of Internal Medicine (2004)[282]

- *Weight: −20.7 pounds versus −10.6 pounds*
- *Plus improved lipid levels and better participant retention*

One hundred and twenty overweight individuals with elevated blood lipids were randomized to a very low-carbohydrate (initially, less than twenty grams of carbohydrates daily) or a low-fat diet. The low-fat group was calorie restricted (five hundred to one thousand calories deficit per day). The study went on for twenty-four weeks.

The study concluded: "Compared with the low-fat diet, the very-low-carb Atkins diet had better participant retention, and greater weight loss −20.7 lbs on average compared to −10.6 lbs. During active

---

282 W. S. Yancy Jr. et al., "A Low-Carbohydrate, Ketogenic Diet versus a low-fat diet to treat obesity and hyperlipidemia," *Annals of Internal Medicine* (2004), http://www.ncbi.nlm. nih.gov/pubmed/15148063.

weight loss, serum triglyceride levels decreased more and HDL choles-terol level increased more with the low-carbohydrate diet."

Six-Month Study Published in the New England Journal of Medicine (2003)[283]

- *Weight: –12.8 pounds versus –4.2 pounds*
- *Improved lipid levels*
- *Improved insulin sensitivity*

One hundred and thirty-two severely obese subjects with a mean BMI of 43 and a high prevalence of diabetes (39%) or the metabolic syndrome (43%) were randomly assigned to a low-carbohydrate diet or a calorie-restricted, low-fat diet for six months. The subjects assigned to the low-carbohydrate diet were instructed to restrict their carbohy-drate intake to thirty grams per day or less. No instruction on restrict-ing total fat intake was provided. Vegetables and fruits with high ratios of fiber to carbohydrates were recommended. The subjects assigned to the low-fat diet received instruction in accordance with the obe-sity-management guidelines of the National Heart, Lung, and Blood Institute, including caloric restriction sufficient to create a deficit of five hundred calories per day, with 30 percent or less of total calories derived from fat.

The study concludes, "Subjects on the low-carb diet lost more weight than those on the low-fat diet mean 12.8 lbs vs. 4.2 lbs and had greater decreases in triglyceride levels. Insulin sensitivity, measured only in subjects without diabetes, also improved more among subjects on the low-carb diet."

---

283 Frederick F. Samaha et al., "A Low-Carbohydrate as Compared with a Low-Fat Diet in Severe Obesity," *New England Journal of Medicine* (2003), http://www.nejm.org/doi/full/10.1056/NEJMoa022637.

Six-Month Study Published in Nutrition and Metabolism (2008)[284]

- *Weight: –24.4 pounds versus –15.2 pounds*
- *Improved lipid levels*
- *Improved glucose levels*
- *Reduced need for medications*

In a twenty-four-week study, eighty-four individuals with obesity and type 2 diabetes were randomized to a low-carbohydrate, ketogenic diet or a low-glycemic-index, reduced-calorie diet (five hundred calories deficit per day).

1. The low-carbohydrate group lost more weight—24.4 pounds versus 15.2 pounds.
2. The blood sugar measurement of hemoglobin A1c went down by 1.5 percent in the low-carbohydrate group versus 0.5 percent in the low-glycemic-index group. (Hemoglobin A1c measures the average blood sugar level over the past two to three months.)
3. HDL cholesterol increased in the low-carbohydrate group (5.6 mg/dL).
4. Diabetes medications were either reduced or eliminated in 95.2 percent of the low-carbohydrate group versus 62 percent in the low-glycemic-index group.

---

284 Eric C. Westman et al., "The Effect of a Low-Carbohydrate, Ketogenic Diet versus a Low-Glycemic Index Diet on Glycemic Control in Type 2 Diabetes Mellitus,." *Nutrition & Metabolism* (2008), http://www.ncbi.nlm.nih.gov/pmc/articles/PMC2633336/.

Six-Month Study Published in the International
Journal of Obesity (1999)[285]

- *Weight: –19.6 pounds versus –11.2 pounds*

Sixty-five overweight subjects were randomized to either a high-carbohydrate, low-protein group with a ratio of carbohydrates to fat to protein of 58:30:12 or a moderate-carbohydrate, high-protein group with a ratio of 45:30:25 for six months. Both groups ate the controlled proportions ad libitum. The higher-protein group lost nearly twice as much weight (–19.6 lb. vs. –11.2 lb.). Both groups attained more than 90 percent of their total weight loss in the first fourteen weeks out of the twenty-six-week trial.

The study concludes that replacement of some dietary carbohydrate by protein in ad libitum fat-reduced diets for treatment of obesity improves mean weight loss. Slight improvements in blood lipids were also observed.

Twelve-Month Study Published in the New
England Journal of Medicine (2003)[286]

- *Weight loss was significantly greater in short-term, but only modestly better after one year.*

Sixty-three individuals were randomized to either a calorie-restricted diet based on the Department of Agriculture Food Guide Pyramid. This diet had a carbohydrate to fat to protein ratio of 60:25:15. The other diet studied was a very low-carbohydrate diet, unrestricted in fats

285 A. R. Skov et al., "Randomized Trial on Protein vs. Carbohydrate in Ad Libitum Fat Reduced Diet for the Treatment of Obesity," *International Journal of Obesity* (1999), http://www.ncbi.nlm.nih.gov/pubmed/10375057.
286 Gary D. Foster et al., "A Randomized Trial of a Low-Carbohydrate Diet for Obesity," *New England Journal of Medicine* (2003), http://www.nejm.org/doi/full/10.1056/NEJMoa022207#t=articleMethods.

and proteins and based on *Dr. Atkins' New Diet Revolution.* The study went on for twelve months.

The study concludes,

Subjects on the low-carb diet lost significantly more weight 6.8% of total body weight, compared to the subjects on the conventional diet, who lost 2.7% at 3 months, and 7.0% vs. 3.2% at 6 months, but the difference in weight loss 4.4% vs. 2.5% was not statistically significant at 12 months. The lack of a statistically significant difference between the groups at one year is most likely due to the difficulty of long-term adherence to the low-carb Atkins diet. As compared with the conventional diet, the low-carb diet was associated with a greater improvement in some risk factors for coronary heart disease (serum triglycerides and serum HDL cholesterol), but not others (blood pressure, insulin sensitivity, and serum LDL cholesterol). This study in particular showed that improvements in cardiovascular-disease risk markers are stable beyond the point at which the diets become similar and weight loss differences become small.

Twelve-Month Study Published in the Journal of the American Medical Association (2007)[287]

- *Weight: –10.3 pounds versus –3.5/5.7/4.9 pounds*

In a study comparing four weight-loss diets representing a spectrum of low- to high-carbohydrate intake for effects on weight loss and related metabolic variables, 311 overweight or obese nondiabetic, premenopausal women were randomly assigned to follow either the Atkins (very low carbohydrate), Zone (moderate to low carbohydrate),

---

287 Christopher D. Gardner et al., "Comparison of the Atkins, Zone, Ornish, and Learn Diets for Change in Weight and Related Risk Factors among Overweight Premenopausal Women: The A to Z Weight Loss Study," *Journal of the American Medical Association* (2007), http://jama.jamanetwork.com/article.aspx?articleid=205916.

LEARN (high carbohydrate and low fat, based on national guidelines), or the Ornish (very high carbohydrate) diet for twelve months.

The study concludes, "The Atkins group on average lost roughly double the weight each of the other groups, and experienced more favorable overall metabolic effects at 12 months –4.7 kg (–10.3 lb.). Weight loss was not statistically different among the Zone, LEARN, and Ornish groups. Zone –1.6 kg (–3.5 lb.), LEARN –2.6 kg (–5.7 lb.), and Ornish –2.2 kg (–4.9 lb.)."

*Twelve-Month Study Published in the
Journal of Nutrition (2009)*[288]

- *Fat loss: 16.1 pounds versus 11.7 pounds*
- *Improved triglycerides and HDL*

One hundred and thirty obese middle-aged subjects were randomized to two energy-restricted diets. The first option was a high-protein diet with a five hundred calorie per day deficit and a carbohydrate to fat to protein ratio of 40:30:30. The second option was a high-carbohydrate diet with a ratio of 55:30:15.

Both groups made the bulk of their body-composition improvements in the first four months:

- *Weight reduction: high-protein –8.2 kg; high-carbohydrate –7.0 kg*
- *Fat loss: high-protein –5.6 kg; high-carbohydrate –4.6 kg*

During the next eight months, improvements were minimal:

- *Weight reduction: high-protein –2.2 kg; high-carbohydrate –1.4 kg*
- *Fat loss: high-protein –1.7 kg; high-carbohydrate –0.7 kg*

---

288   D. K. Layman et al., "A Moderate-Protein Diet Produces Sustained Weight Loss and Long-Term Changes in Body Composition and Blood Lipids in Obese Adults," *Journal of Nutrition* (2009), http://jn.nutrition.org/content/139/3/514.long.

The cumulative results for twelve months are as follows:

- *Weight reduction: high-protein –10.4 kg; high-carbohydrate –8.4 kg*
- *Fat loss: high-protein –7.3 kg (16.1 lb.); high-carbohydrate –5.3 kg (11.7 lb.)*

At four months, the high-protein group had lost 22 percent more fat mass than the high-carbohydrate group. At twelve months, the high-protein group had more participants complete the study (64% vs. 45%) with greater improvement in body composition; however, weight loss did not differ significantly between the groups (–10.4 kg vs. –8.4 kg). The high-carbohydrate diet reduced serum cholesterol and LDL cholesterol compared with the high-protein diet at four months, but the effect did not remain at twelve months. The high-protein group sustained favorable effects on serum triacylglycerol (TAG), HDL cholesterol (HDL-C), and TAG:HDL-C compared with the high-carbohydrate group at four and twelve months.

The study concludes, "The high-protein diet was more effective for fat-mass loss and body composition improvement during initial weight loss and long-term maintenance (38 percent greater fat-loss at twelve months) and produced sustained reductions in serum triacylglycerol TAG and increases in HDL-C compared with the high-carb diet; however, the bulk of the fat loss was attained in the first four months."

META-ANALYSES

The above sampling of studies can be somewhat justifiably depicted as "cherry-picked" studies that fit my agenda. In contrast, meta-analysis lumps together all relevant studies that meet the criteria of the analysis. Here is a summary of six recent meta-analyses. The reason they have different results and conclusions is because they have different inclusion criteria.

Meta-Analysis of Seventy-Four Studies: "Effects of
Higher- versus Lower-Protein Diets on Health Outcomes:
A Systematic Review and Meta-Analysis."[289]

This meta-analysis concludes, "(a) Higher-protein diets improve adiposity, blood pressure and triglyceride levels, but these effects are small. (b) Translated to an effect at three months, the meta-analysis shows a greater weight loss of 1.21 kg (2.66 lb.), a greater decrease in BMI (–0.51 kg/m2) and a greater loss in waist circumference –1.66 cm (0.66 inches) in higher-protein compared with lower-protein diets."

Meta-Analysis of Fifteen Studies: "Long-Term Effects
of Low-Fat Diets Either Low or High in Protein on
Cardiovascular and Metabolic Risk Factors: A
Systematic Review and Meta-Analysis."[290]

In contrast, this meta-analysis only includes long-term studies of no less than one year. In this study most of the benefits of the high-protein diet are considered *insignificant* at twelve months: improved weight loss is only 0.86 pounds more, fat loss is 1.3 pounds more, and triglyceride reduction is 2.87 mg/dL greater. Only the improvement of fasting insulin (–0.71 µIU/ml) was considered significant.

Considering that 9.3 percent of adults have diabetes and another 32 percent have prediabetes, the fasting insulin benefits are of relevance to a large portion of the population.

Upon closer investigation of this analysis, I realized that most of the "long-term studies" it includes are actually only three-month diets, with a checkup a year later. The study's conclusion that long-term, high-protein diets have no significant benefits appears to be a distortion

---

289 N. Santesso et al., "Effects of Higher- versus Lower-Protein Diets on Health Outcomes: A Systematic Review and Meta-Analysis," *European Journal of Clinical Nutrition* (2012), http://www.nature.com/ejcn/journal/v66/n7/full/ejcn201237a.html.
290 Lukas Schwingshackl and Georg Hoffmann, "Long-Term Effects of Low-Fat Diets Either Low or High in Protein on Cardiovascular and Metabolic Risk Factors: A Systematic Review and Meta-Analysis," *Nutrition Journal* (2013), http://www.biomedcentral.com/content/pdf/1475-2891-12-48.pdf.

of the reality that benefits of the three-month diets eventually become "insignificant" when not adhered to long enough.

There is also a confusion of two separate issues: short-term fat loss and long-term maintenance of reduced fat mass. Low-carbohydrate, high-protein diets work the best for short-term fat loss. Even though such diets are insufficient for solving the long-term maintenance of fat loss, their short-term value shouldn't be ignored. But beyond the short-term fat-loss benefits, there are also the long-term benefits for those with tendencies toward high blood sugar levels, as mentioned above.

Meta-Analysis of Forty-Eight Randomized Controlled Studies: "The Effects of High Protein Diets on Thermogenesis, Satiety and Weight Loss: A Critical Review."[291]

This meta-analysis included studies that compare relatively high-protein diets to lower-protein diets. Most studies find that higher protein diets

- **Increase energy expenditure:** All six of the studies that assess the thermic effect of food as a percentage of ingested energy report greater energy expenditure for the higher-protein versus the lower-protein diet.
- **Increase subjective ratings of satiety:** Of the fourteen studies evaluating satiety, eleven report that a protein preload significantly increases subjective ratings of satiety; the remaining three studies report no difference.
- **Decrease subsequent energy intake:** Of the fifteen studies evaluating subsequent energy intake, eight report a significant decrease in energy intake after a higher versus lower protein preload; the other seven studies reported no significant differences.

---

291 T. L. Halton and F. B. Hu, "The Effects of High Protein Diets on Thermogenesis, Satiety and Weight Loss: A Critical Review," *Journal of the American College of Nutrition* (2004), http://www.colorado.edu/intphys/Class/IPHY3700_Greene/pdfs/discussionEssay/thermogenesisSatiety/HaltonProtein2004.pdf.

- **Increase weight loss:** Of the fifteen studies evaluating total weight loss, seven report a significantly greater weight loss with a higher-protein diet. Five of these studies were of longer duration (six months or more), two were of shorter duration (a few weeks), and eight report no significant difference in weight loss.
- **Increase fat loss:** Of the ten studies evaluating total fat loss, most find greater fat loss with the high-protein diets in comparison to the lower-protein diets, but only three studies find this difference to be statistically significant.

The study's conclusion is that "higher protein diets might increase weight loss in the short term, but further longer term research is required before definitive conclusions can be drawn."

Meta-Analysis That Includes Randomized Clinical Trials with an Intervention/Follow-Up of At Least Twenty-Four Weeks: "Long-Term Efficacy of High-Protein Diets: A Systematic Review."[292]

This meta-analysis looks at eight studies that meet the inclusion criteria. It finds that in the studies, the average weight loss of participants following the high-protein diet was 6.3 kilograms and in the standard diet was 5.0 kilograms. Although half of the studies show a higher weight loss with a high-protein diet, three out of four studies with the longest intervention show no statistical difference in weight loss. This systematic review observes that the *long-term* effect of high-protein diets is neither consistent nor conclusive.

---

292 M. Lepe, M. Bacardí Gascón, and A. Jiménez Cruz, "Long-Term Efficacy of High-Protein Diets: A Systematic Review," *Nutrición hospitalaria* (2011), http://www.ncbi.nlm.nih.gov/pubmed/22411369.

Systematic Review of Thirteen Studies Comparing Low-Carb versus Low-Fat Diets: "Systematic Review of Randomized Controlled Trials of Low-Carbohydrate vs. Low-Fat/Low-Calorie Diets in the Management of Obesity and Its Comorbidities."[293]
This review looks at studies from 2000 to 2007, excluding

- seventy-one studies that are nonrandomized or controlled trials,
- fifty studies in which subjects did not receive appropriate treatment,
- thirty-six studies of less than six months,
- fourteen studies in which the carbohydrate content of the "low-carbohydrate" diet was too high,
- six studies in which the subjects were under eighteen,
- five studies where the participants were not human, and
- five studies in which participants have a BMI of less than 28.

The review finds that the low-carbohydrate, high-protein diet surpasses the control diets in weight loss by four kilograms at the six-month mark but only by one kilogram by the twelve-month mark.

293 M Hession et al., "Systematic Review of Randomized Controlled Trials of Low-Carbohydrate vs. Low-Fat/Low-Calorie Diets in the Management of Obesity and Its Comorbidities," *Obesity Reviews* (2009), http://onlinelibrary.wiley.com/doi/10.1111/j.1467-789X.2008.00518.x/pdf.

*A Meta-Analysis Investigating whether Individuals
Assigned to a Very Low-Carbohydrate, Ketogenic Diet
Achieve Better Long-Term Body Weight and Cardiovascular
Risk-Factor Management Than Individuals Assigned to
a Conventional Low-Fat Diet: "Very-Low-Carbohydrate
Ketogenic Diet v. Low-Fat Diet for Long-Term Weight Loss:
A Meta-Analysis of Randomised Controlled Trials."[294]*

A very low-carbohydrate, ketogenic diet (VLCKD) is a diet that allows individuals to consume no more than fifty grams of carbohydrates per day. A low-fat diet is a restricted-energy diet where individuals consume less than 30 percent of their energy from fat. A total of thirteen studies met the inclusion/exclusion criteria. Individuals assigned to a VLCKD showed significant: decreased body weight, triglycerides, and diastolic blood pressure, with increased HDL-C and LDL-C.

*Meta-analysis of seventeen studies: "Dietary Intervention
for Overweight and Obese Adults: Comparison of Low-
Carbohydrate and Low-Fat Diets. A Meta-Analysis"[295]*

A most recent (Oct. 2015) meta-analysis of seventeen randomized controlled trials from 8 weeks to 24 months in duration, comparing low carbohydrate (≤120gm carbohydrates/day) and low fat diet (≤30% energy from fat/day) concludes: Compared with low fat diet, low carbohydrate was associated with significantly greater reduction in weight and significantly lower predicted risk of atherosclerotic cardiovascular disease events. The probability of greater weight loss associated with low carbohydrate was >99%, and the reduction in predicted ASCVD risk favoring low carbohydrate was >98%.

---

294 N. B. Bueno et al., "Very-Low-Carbohydrate Ketogenic Diet v. Low-Fat Diet for Long-Term Weight Loss: A Meta-Analysis of Randomised Controlled Trials," *British Journal of Nutrition* (2013), http://www.ncbi.nlm.nih.gov/pubmed/23651522.
295 J. Sackner-Bernstein, D. Kanter, Sanjay Kaul, "Dietary Intervention for Overweight and Obese Adults: Comparison of Low-Carbohydrate and Low-Fat Diets. A Meta-Analysis", PLoS One, (Oct. 2015), http://journals.plos.org/plosone/article?id=10.1371/journal.pone.0139817.

CONCLUSION

It appears that the low-carbohydrate, high-protein diet clearly fares the best up to six months in regard to improving the conditions of the metabolic syndrome (e.g., waistline, triglycerides, HDLs, blood pressure, and blood sugar), whereas with longer-term use, the advantages diminish, with the exception of lowered blood sugar levels that continue even long term.

While some dietitians reject the use of low-carbohydrate diets because they only recommend diets that work long term, I explained in part I how fat loss is most successful for many people by using short-term diets that reduce body fat moderately, then shifting to a maintenance diet until the body has accustomed itself to the lower weight, and then repeatedly switching between short-term fat loss and maintenance diets. We investigate this method further in the last chapter.

15

Pros and Cons of Some of the Most Popular Diets

Each of these diets works for some people but not for others. By examining the pros and cons of each diet, we can extract something instructive and positive from all of them. Some diets are based on phases that change after a few days, weeks, or months; other diets are continuous without any distinct phases. Some of the diets entail risks and negative repercussions. This chapter summarizes and examines the pros and cons of the following diets:

1. The Atkins Diet (Dr. Robert C. Atkins): four phases
2. Eat to Live (Dr. Joel Fuhrman)
3. The Paleo Diet (Dr. Loren Cordain)
4. The Venice Nutrition Program—Body Confidence (Mark Macdonald)
5. The Dukan Diet (Dr. Pierre Dukan): four phases
6. The South Beach Diet (Dr. Arthur Agatston): three phases
7. The Zone (Dr. Barry Sears)
8. The Fast Diet (Dr. Michael Mosley and Mimi Spencer)
9. The No-Fad Diet (American Heart Association)

THE ATKINS DIET
Dr. Robert C. Atkins

The Atkins diet consists of four phases.

Phase 1: Induction
This two-week phase (it can be longer) involves fast weight loss via minimal carbohydrate intake (no more than twenty grams, primarily from salad greens). Lack of fiber can be compensated for with a tablespoon of psyllium husks, ground flaxseed, or wheat bran.

Phase 2: Ongoing Weight Loss
This phase moves to a slower weight-loss plan by graduating to a slightly normalized carbohydrate intake. Each week, daily carbohydrate intake is increased by five grams until the individual reaches the "critical carbohydrate level for losing." This level is discovered when weight loss stops, at which point carbohydrate intake is reduced to a level where ongoing weight loss can continue.

Phase 3: Premaintenance
Carbohydrate levels are increased again; however, at this stage, when the dieter is within five to ten pounds of his or her target weight, the objective is to lose these last pounds slowly, at a rate of only one pound per week. The reason for this phase is to "train" for the final Lifetime Maintenance phase.

Phase 4: Lifetime Maintenance
During this phase, dieters learn how to restrict themselves to maintain a healthy weight. By the time they get to this phase, dieters have learned what their personal "critical carbohydrate level for maintenance" is. They are encouraged to restrict themselves to this level for life.

The Atkins Diet Induces Fat Loss by Ketosis

Ketosis is the metabolic state when most of the body's energy supply comes from *ketone bodies,* in contrast to a state of *glycolysis,* where *glucose* provides most of the energy. Most cells in the body can use both glucose and ketone bodies for fuel, and during ketosis when most of the body's energy supply comes from ketone bodies, free fatty acids and glucose synthesis (gluconeogenesis) fuel the remainder.

During the usual overnight fast, the body's metabolism naturally switches into ketosis and switches back to glycolysis after a carbohydrate-rich meal. Longer-term ketosis is attained by fasting or abstaining from carbohydrates. When in glycolysis (the body being fueled primarily by glucose) as opposed to ketosis, higher levels of insulin promote storage of body fat and block release of fat from adipose tissues, while in ketosis, fat reserves are readily released and consumed. The Atkins diet is a very low-carbohydrate diet that aims for longer-term ketosis, the body's "fat burning" mode.

Interesting Facts about Ketosis

During the process of lipolysis, lipids are broken down, yielding ketones—a form of usable stored energy that is different from glucose. Ketone bodies are three water-soluble molecules that are produced by the liver from fatty acids. The three endogenous ketone bodies are acetone, acetoacetic acid, and beta-hydroxybutyric acid. Two of the three are used as a source of energy in the heart and brain, while the third (acetone) is a degradation breakdown product of acetoacetic acid.

Between 2 and 30 percent of the acetone is excreted from the body. If it is not used for energy or converted to pyruvate, it is removed as waste. This "use it or lose it" factor may contribute to the weight loss found in ketogenic (low-carbohydrate) diets. Acetone cannot be converted back to acetyl-CoA, so it is excreted in the urine or (as a consequence of its high vapor pressure) exhaled unless first converted to pyruvate. Acetone is responsible for the characteristic "sweet and fruity" odor of the breath of persons in ketosis.

Pros of the Atkins Diet

1. The Atkins diet is a fast way to lose weight for most people. Numerous studies show that the very low-carbohydrate diet enables faster weight loss than does any other diet in which the same amount of calories are consumed.
2. It helps lower and stabilize blood sugar levels, and as a result, one's liver produces less cholesterol. Eventually, this diet helps reduce blood pressure levels for people who have problems with high blood pressure.
3. Some find this diet easy because it only restricts carbohydrate intake and doesn't require counting calories of proteins and fats.

Cons of the Atkins Diet

1. It is difficult to get sufficient fiber during the induction phase. This is not critical since the induction phase is not long term; however, even on the maintenance plan, carbohydrates are limited to forty to sixty grams, which makes obtaining sufficient fiber challenging. Most people get less than half the fiber they need—even though their diets include over 50 percent of caloric intake from carbohydrates (roughly 250 grams or more). As fiber is attained only in carbohydrates, reducing them to less than 10 percent of caloric intake is likely to exacerbate the fiber deficiency unless one includes fiber supplements.
2. When dieters suddenly change to a severely restricted carbohydrate intake but remain unrestricted in their protein and fat intake, they will see success in weight loss only if their nature doesn't allow them to eat fats and proteins wildly. But people who love indulging in fats and proteins benefit little

in terms of weight loss by only restricting their carbohydrate intake.

3. Numerous studies conclude that the low-carbohydrate diet produces a greater weight loss than a conventional diet for the first six months, but the differences are not significant at one year.[296, 297, 298]

4. Long-term use of the very low-carbohydrate diet can also lead to raised LDL levels[299]—a risk for heart disease.

5. Even the "Lifetime Maintenance" phase of the Atkins diet is low carb. Atkins recommends forty to sixty grams of carbohydrates per day for the average person (less than 10 percent of total caloric intake!), in contrast with the recommendations of the US Department of Health, in which carbohydrate intake is 45 to 65 percent of caloric intake[300] (this would be approximately three hundred grams of carbohydrates per day for the average person). Many people find this limitation too restrictive and impossible to live with on a permanent basis. Additionally, the body cannot function optimally on such a low proportion of carbohydrates. Atkins does allow ninety grams of carbohydrates or more per day for someone who does vigorous exercise

296   Gary D. Foster et al., "A Randomized Trial of a Low-Carbohydrate Diet for Obesity," *New England Journal of Medicine* (2003), http://www.nejm.org/doi/full/10.1056/NEJMoa022207#t=articleMethods.

297   Christopher D. Gardner et al., "Comparison of the Atkins, Zone, Ornish, and Learn Diets for Change in Weight and Related Risk Factors among Overweight Premenopausal Women: The A to Z Weight Loss Study," *Journal of the American Medical Association* (2007), http://jama.jamanetwork.com/article.aspx?articleid=205916.

298   I. Shai et al., "Weight Loss with a Low-Carbohydrate, Mediterranean, or Low-Fat Diet," *New England Journal of Medicine* (2008), http://www.nejm.org/doi/full/10.1056/NEJMoa0708681.

299   N. B. Bueno et al., "Very-Low-Carbohydrate Ketogenic Diet v. Low-Fat Diet for Long-Term Weight Loss: A Meta-Analysis of Randomised Controlled Trials," *British Journal of Nutrition* (2013), http://www.ncbi.nlm.nih.gov/pubmed/23651522.

300   US Department of Agriculture; US Department of Health and Human Services (www.dietaryguidelines.gov); based on the findings of the Institute of Medicine, *Dietary Reference Intakes*, 1325.

for forty minutes, five days per week, but even ninety grams is extremely low and inhibits athletes from performing their best. Virtually no professional athletes maintain their body weight and perform professionally while on such an extremely low-carbohydrate diet. Insulin speeds up absorption of nutrients, which is why a higher-carbohydrate diet is necessary for athletes to recover from intense workouts.

6. For many people, the ongoing weight-loss phase doesn't work. At some point (far before the target weight is reached), the metabolism slows drastically. When fat mass is reduced without a matching reduction in fat cell numbers, fat cells release less leptin, which in turn slows metabolism, increases efficiency in calorie absorption, and drives up hunger. Low leptin levels also weaken one's immune system, making one susceptible to infection. Many people "hit a wall"—for which Atkins has no solutions. When the dieter gets fed up with such a restricted low-carbohydrate diet and begins increasing his or her carbohydrate intake, there is a likelihood of a weight rebound, often causing more weight to be gained back than was lost.

Criticism of the Atkins Diet

The Atkins book gives the impression that a person either burns fat as fuel or burns stored sugars as fuel, as opposed to using both fuel sources simultaneously. This is far from the truth.

Dr. Atkins's diet revolution suggests,[301] "If you're not in lipolysis, you're in glucosis. The two fuel sources are your body's alternative, completely parallel options for energy metabolism. This terminology has helped many of my patients convince their doctors or dietitians that Atkins was the right path."

---

301 Robert C. Atkins, *Dr. Atkins' New Diet Revolution*, New York, HarperCollins Publishers, (2002), 59.

Most readers interpret this and similar statements of Atkins as saying that the body is either being fueled by burning stored glucose or by burning stored fats, and they mistakenly assume that the body can't be fueled by both sources at the same time.

First of all, *"glucosis"* is a word that exists only in Atkins's book. The word he is actually referring to is *glycolysis*. Both the words *glycolysis* and *lipolysis* are composed of two parts: *glyco* and *lysis* and *lipo* and *lysis. Lysis* means "break down." *Glyco* refers to stored sugars—glucose stored as glycogen. And *lipo* refers to stored fats, or lipids.

In truth, concerning the body's sources of fuel, when the blood sugar level drops, the body maintains energy levels by *both* lipolysis and glycolysis (breaking down both stored fats and sugars).

The state of *ketosis* occurs when lipolysis is the dominant source of energy. While it is true that a person is either in a state of ketosis or a state of glycolysis, this only means that one process or the other is *dominant*. For example, if 70 percent of energy is coming from the process of lipolysis and 30 percent from glycolysis, the person is in a state of ketosis (lipolysis dominant). It doesn't have to be 100 percent against 0 percent, and it rarely is.

The only way to effect lipolysis, or burning stored fat, *exclusively*—without glycolysis, or burning stored glucose—is if all reserves of glycogen (stored glucose) are depleted. True, the body will employ lipolysis as a method for providing energy at a faster rate (in other words, it will burn fat faster) when the option of providing energy via glycolysis is not available; nevertheless, it is a mistake to think that lipolysis can't occur at all as long as glycolysis is an option. In fact, in normal, healthy people who are on not on calorie-restricted diets and eat normal amounts of carbohydrates, lipolysis is the dominant provider of energy when sleeping, especially as the night continues, the glycogen reserves go down, and catabolic hormones such as cortisol rise. An additional method of speeding the lipolysis process (as recommended by Maimonides) is to do aerobic exercise in the morning before breakfast, when cortisol is at its daily peak.

EAT TO LIVE
Dr. Joel Fuhrman

Dr. Fuhrman's focus is on the quality of the food we digest. He recommends eating foods that are high in nutrients, high in fiber, low in calories, low in protein, and low in fat. And he suggests avoiding animal products (including meat, fish, eggs, and even dairy) and grains.

Pros of Eat to Live
1. What is good about Dr. Fuhrman's diet is his emphasis on fruits and vegetables, particularly fresh vegetables, as well as legumes, nuts, and seeds—foods that are high in nutrients and fiber. Most people are eating too many processed foods of high carbohydrates and unhealthy fats with little nutrients and fiber.
2. Avoiding meat, fish, dairy, and all processed foods, as well as severely limiting grains, while surviving solely on fruits, vegetables, legumes, nuts, and seeds, will naturally lead to calorie reduction, causing weight loss in the short term.

Cons of Eat to Live
1. For most people, the extreme restrictions are not practical; people simply can't adjust to such drastic changes of cutting out both animal products and grains.
2. Dr. Fuhrman recommends[302] consuming less than the USDA RDA minimum of fifty-six grams of protein for male adults and forty-six for women. Such a minimal amount of protein means that all energy must come from carbohydrates and fats. That makes stabilizing blood sugar levels nearly impossible for people with diabetes or prediabetes. Consuming larger

---

302 Joel Fuhrman, *Eat to Live: The Amazing Nutrient-Rich Program for Fast and Sustained Weight Loss*, New York, Little Brown (2011), 39.

quantities of proteins and fats than needed for cellular maintenance enables the extra proteins and fats to serve as fuel, without spiking insulin levels, and is essential for stabilizing blood sugar.

3. This extreme low-protein diet is likely to weaken the immune system[303] and cause a loss of muscle. The RDA of protein is a minimum for protein homeostasis—*when the body is not running on a caloric deficit.* When reducing calories and running on a deficit, the body burns stored fats and *proteins* to generate glucose. If there are insufficient proteins in the diet for homeostasis, the body literally consumes muscle to produce energy. According to *The Textbook of Medical Physiology,*[304] at least sixty to seventy-five grams of protein is recommended for the average adult—the RDA being insufficient. Certainly athletes and those serious about resistance training need much more protein than Dr. Fuhrman's diet provides. Such a low-protein diet makes it impossible to recuperate from workouts and build muscle.

4. Low-calorie diets inevitably slow down a person's metabolic rate—causing the body to conserve energy and burn fewer calories. Losing muscle mass due to the extreme low-protein content also lowers the metabolic rate. According to numerous studies (see previous chapter), restricted-calorie diets that are high in carbohydrates burn less fat than low-carbohydrate diets and increase hunger.

5. In the Eat to Live diet, the percentage of calories is approximately 80 percent carbohydrates. For diabetics, this is too liberal. As healthy as fruits are, they raise the blood sugar level, and too much of a good thing is a danger for diabetics. A meta-analysis of 15 *long-term* studies show that low-carbohydrate diets

---

303   Institute of Medicine, *Dietary Reference Intakes,* 608–609.
304   Guyton and Hall, *Textbook of Medical Physiology,* Saunders (2011), 835.

lower glucose and insulin levels and are better for diabetics/pre-diabetics than regular or high-carbohydrate diets.[305]

6. Many people who succeed in losing weight in the short term with this diet get fed up with the restrictions and hunger and go back to eating normally—healthy meat, fish, dairy, and grains—not to mention occasionally snacking on junk food when their schedule is too busy. As Eat to Live offers no long term-solutions to reduce fat cell number, increase leptin sensitivity, and maintain a healthy metabolic rate, there is a likelihood of gaining back all the lost weight and more.

Criticism of Eat to Live

Concerning protein, Dr. Fuhrman references numerous studies linking consumption of animal proteins (meat, fish, eggs, and dairy products) to various cancers, heart disease, and the loss of calcium and other essential minerals, leading to weakening of the bones. The problem is that none of the references cite controlled studies but rather population comparisons. Correlations between animal protein consumption and his list of illnesses do not qualify as proof of cause.

Despite the fact that he is correct that high amounts of protein in the diet are closely associated with increased urinary-calcium excretion, nevertheless, the majority of epidemiological studies have shown that long-term high-protein intake increases bone-mineral density and reduces bone-fracture incidence. The reason is that the beneficial effects of protein, such as increasing intestinal calcium absorption, circulating IGF-I, and lowering serum parathyroid hormone, sufficiently offset any negative effects of the acid load of protein on bone health.[306]

---

305 Lukas Schwingshackl and Georg Hoffmann, "Long-Term Effects of Low-Fat Diets Either Low or High in Protein on Cardiovascular and Metabolic Risk Factors: A Systematic Review and Meta-Analysis," *Nutrition Journal* (2013), http://www.biomedcentral.com/content/pdf/1475-2891-12-48.pdf.

306 J. J. Cao and F. H. Nielsen, "Acid Diet (High-Meat Protein) Effects on Calcium Metabolism and Bone Health," *Current Opinion in Clinical Nutrition and Metabolic Care* (2010), http://www.ncbi.nlm.nih.gov/pubmed/20717017.

In *Eat to Live*,[307] Dr. Fuhrman attempts to demonstrate a correlation between animal-protein intake and hip-fracture rate, and he quotes a study listing the animal-protein intake of sixteen countries and their hip-fracture rate. While a few countries do show the correlation that he points to, other countries demonstrate just the opposite. For example, in Israel, animal-protein intake is 42.5 grams per day, and the hip-fracture rate is 93.2 per one hundred thousand people—a high hip-fracture rate. Spain and the Netherlands have a higher animal-protein intake yet a *lower* hip-fracture rate; in fact, the hip-fracture rate of Spain is less than half of that of Israel! Even Ireland, with a significantly higher animal-protein intake than Israel, at 61.4 grams per day compared to Israel's 42.5, has a significantly lower hip-fracture rate of seventy-six per one hundred thousand. Sweden, with an animal-protein intake of less than sixty grams per day, has a higher hip-fracture rate than Finland, Ireland, the United States, and New Zealand, despite the fact that all these countries have animal-protein intakes of over sixty grams per day. In fact, New Zealand's animal-protein intake is nearly eighty grams per day, 30 percent more than that of Sweden, yet Sweden's hip-fracture rate is 187.8 and New Zealand's is 119! Despite Ireland's having a higher animal-protein intake than Sweden, Ireland's hip-fracture rate is a mere seventy-six, compared to Sweden's 187.8. Yet Dr. Fuhrman will have his readers believe that this study proves that increased animal protein causes calcium loss? And it is not even a controlled study. Actually, from this study, we can conclude just the opposite—that there is no correlation between animal-protein intake and calcium loss; rather, the varying rate of hip fracture between countries is due to other reasons.

Controlled studies have yet to prove any correlation between moderate animal-protein consumption and diseases, except in the case of people with kidney problems, where eating too much protein strains the kidneys further. Also, for some individuals, eating exorbitant amounts of animal protein can lead to loss of calcium.

---

307 Fuhrman, *Eat to Live*, New York, Little Brown (2011), 105.

The reason that drawing conclusions from population studies is not reliable is because there are thousands of variables that can be the actual cause of the higher rates of cancer, heart disease, and the like. For example, air pollution or water pollution is different for each population and locality, and people's different lifestyles and levels of physical exertion can also account for health differences among different populations (city folk sit at desks, country folk work on farms). As such, it is unscientific to jump to the conclusion that specifically the dietary differences (or one specific dietary difference) between populations account for all their health differences.

Furthermore, putting all dairy products into one basket of ill health is misleading. Some cheeses are high in saturated fats and cholesterol, while others are not. Similarly, there are lean meats and fatty cuts. Meat, fish, eggs, and dairy products that are of good nutritional quality supply complete proteins together with other nutrients—calcium in dairy, iron in meat, and fish oils are extremely beneficial. When eaten in moderation, animal proteins are very beneficial to one's health.

Moreover, causing people to fear that eating healthy animal proteins will give them cancer and heart disease is counterproductive. Competitive athletes need animal proteins to develop their strength. Cutting out meat, fish, eggs, and dairy in such an extreme manner as Dr. Fuhrman recommends will not only limit the success of athletes but also weaken most people as well as unnecessarily restrict their diets in a manner that is difficult to maintain.

The Atkins diet has proven that replacing carbohydrates with fat and protein has helped thousands of people to stabilize blood sugar and lose weight (see previous chapter for details from many studies).

Healthy proteins are satisfying and filling and are also the major structural component of all cells in the body, including body organs, bones, hair, and skin. When broken down into amino acids, proteins are used as precursors to nucleic acid, coenzymes, hormones, immune response, cellular repair, and other molecules that are essential for life. Additionally, protein is needed to form blood cells. And extra protein that is not needed as protein is used by the body as fuel without causing high blood sugar; rather, additional protein helps stabilize blood sugar.

Concerning fat, Dr. Fuhrman writes, "Fat is an appetite stimulant."[308] Dr. Fuhrman brings no sources or studies to back up this claim. One study concludes just the opposite: "Laboratory-based studies investigating physiological effects of fat have demonstrated that the direct exposure of receptors in the oral cavity and small intestine to fat, specifically fatty acids (FAs), induces potent effects on gastrointestinal (GI) motility and gut peptide secretion that favor the suppression of appetite and energy intake."[309]

Concerning wheat, Dr. Fuhrman writes, "Wheat grown on American soil is not a nutrient-dense food to begin with."[310]

Actually, whole grains are an excellent source of fiber, B vitamins, antioxidants, and minerals and have a modest percentage of protein as well. And even if grains do supply a lot of carbohydrates together with these nutrients, carbohydrates are not the devil incarnate. They are an important macronutrient that is very beneficial to our health when eaten in appropriate amounts. More active people need more carbohydrates, and ingesting moderate amounts at the right time of day (three to five hours after waking up in the morning) enables us to function at our best throughout the day. When someone wants to build muscle, the ingestion of larger quantities of carbohydrates increases insulin, which speeds up nutrient intake, enabling faster recovery and muscle building.

---

308 Fuhrman, *Eat to Live*, New York, Little Brown (2011), 44.

309 Little and Feinle-Bisset, "Effects of Dietary Fat **on Appetite and Energy Intake in Health And Obesity—Oral and Gastrointestinal Sensory Contributions**," *Physiology & Behavior* (2011), http://www.ncbi.nlm.nih.gov/pubmed/21596051.

310 Fuhrman, *Eat to Live*, New York, Little Brown (2011), 39.

THE PALEO DIET
Dr. Loren Cordain

The word *paleo* means "prehistoric." The idea of the Paleo diet is to mimic the diet that evolutionists theorize prehistoric humans ate, based on the *assumption* that the body is genetically adapted to function best according to the diet that it survived on over millions of years.

According to these theorists, sixty million years ago, the earliest primates subsisted mainly on fruit, leaves, and insects: humans started using tools and fire 2.6 million years ago and moved to a hunter-gatherer diet. These theorists assume that the body is genetically best adapted to a hunter-gatherer diet, to the exclusion of diets that include grains, legumes, and dairy, which they assume only became part of the human diet ten thousand years ago, when agriculture became a primary method of attaining food.

Dr. Loren Cordain's diet recommendations are as follows:

1. Eat all the lean meats, fish, and seafood you can.
2. Eat all the fruits and nonstarchy vegetables you can.
3. Focus on a diet with a net-alkaline load.
4. Eat foods high in potassium and low in sodium (no salt).
5. Moderate consumption of oils from olive, avocado, and flaxseed.
6. Moderate consumption of artificial sweeteners, caffeine, and alcohol.
7. Moderate consumption nuts and dried fruits.
8. Do not eat grains.
9. Do not eat legumes.
10. Do not eat starchy vegetables such as potatoes, sweet potatoes, or yams.
11. Do not eat dairy products.
12. Do not eat processed foods.
13. Do not eat candy, honey, or sugar.
14. He recommends (pg 24) the following macronutrient division (percentage of calories):

Fats	28–47 percent
Carbohydrates	22–40 percent
Proteins	19–35 percent

Pros of the Paleo Diet

1. By excluding grains, legumes, starchy vegetables, dairy, processed foods, and sugar from their diet, most people will consume fewer calories and thereby lose weight in the short term. Despite the restrictions, the diet includes sufficient macro- and micronutrients for maintaining health.

2. Our bodies need far more potassium than sodium, but the typical US diet is just the opposite: Americans average about 3,300 milligrams of sodium per day, about 75 percent of which comes from processed foods, while only getting about 2,900 milligrams of potassium daily. Sodium and potassium have opposite effects on heart health: high salt intake increases blood pressure, which can lead to heart disease, while high potassium intake can help relax blood vessels and excrete the sodium and decrease blood pressure. Therefore, Dr. Cordain's recommendation concerning salt and potassium is on target.

3. Regarding the problem of consuming too much unhealthy saturated fat when including meat in one's diet, Dr. Cordain raises a good point: "The meat of grain-fed livestock is vastly at odds with that of wild animals. A 100 gram serving of T-bone beefsteak gives you a walloping 9.1 grams of saturated fat whereas a comparable piece of bison roast yields on 0.9 grams of saturated fat."[311] Actually, we don't have to go back so far as prehistoric times to reach the era when most of the meat consumed by humans was free range. Just 150 years ago, that was the norm. However, his emphasis to purchase leaner free-ranging meats is on target.

---

311 Loren Cordain, *The Paleo Diet: Lose Weight and Get Healthy by Eating the Foods You Were Designed to Eat*, New York, NY: Houghton Mifflin Harcourt (2011), 15.

Cons of the Paleo Diet

1. Whole grains, legumes, and many low-fat dairy products are excellent sources of nutrition—dietary fiber, protein, carbohydrates, vitamins, and minerals. Except for individuals who have allergies to these foods or difficulty digesting them, these foods are beneficial and healthful when not overeaten, contributing to a balanced, healthy diet. Food variety is important, as each food contributes something unique for the body to utilize, and the Paleo diet unreasonably limits this variety, placing unnecessary stress on the dieter.

2. The Paleo diet doesn't provide any advice on reducing the number of fat cells or improving leptin sensitivity, which are necessary for long-term fat reduction.

Criticism of the Paleo Diet

1. The presumption that total avoidance of grains, legumes, and dairy products will make you healthy and fit like a prehistoric hunter is incorrect. Avoiding processed foods, sugar, and salt is not unique to the Paleo diet; neither is the recommendation to get exercise unique. What is unique to his diet is the total avoidance of grains, legumes, and dairy products.

   Dr. Cordain attempts to convince people that the unique qualities of the Paleo diet (total avoidance of grains, legumes, and dairy products) make you healthy. In his words, "Descriptions of hunter gatherers by early European explorers and adventurers showed these people to be healthy, fit, strong, and vivacious. These same characteristics can be yours when you follow the dietary and exercise principles I have laid out in the Paleo Diet."[312]

   Prehistoric hunters also didn't use modern laundry detergent and toothbrushes. So should we avoid those too? It's more practical and realistic to mimic the diets and lifestyles of today's

---

312 Ibid., 6.

world-champion athletes—professional football and basketball stars, professional boxers and wrestlers, Olympic track stars, weight lifting champions, and marathon runners. They all eat grains, legumes, and dairy, and they would not have been as successful had they not.

2. The relevance and value of an alkaline diet is unsubstantiated. Concerning Dr. Cordain's recommendation to focus on a diet with a net-alkaline load, I don't see the relevance to the diet of the theorized prehistoric man. Grains, legumes, meat, fish, and eggs are all acidic, while fruits and vegetables are alkaline. Depending upon the location and the season, hunter-gatherers would sometimes have had a more acidic diets and other times a more alkaline diet.

Dr. Cordain adheres to a new, popular, but unsubstantiated theory that it is in our best interest to eat foods that are more alkaline than acidic so that we end up with an overall alkaline load in our body. This supposedly protects us from the diseases of modern civilization, whereas eating a diet with a net-acid load will make us vulnerable to everything from cancer to osteoporosis. A meta-analysis of clinical trials concludes that there is no evidence that increasing the diet acid load promotes skeletal bone-mineral loss or osteoporosis.[313]

3. The inclusion of wine in the Paleo Diet is hypocritical. Dr. Cordain writes, "Numerous scientific studies suggest that moderate alcohol consumption significantly reduces the risk of dying from heart disease and other illnesses. Wine in particular, when consumed in moderation has been shown to have many beneficial health effects."[314]

---

313   T. R. Fenton et al., "Meta-Analysis of the Effect of the Acid-Ash Hypothesis of Osteoporosis on Calcium Balance," *Journal of Bone and Mineral Research* (2009), http://www.ncbi.nlm.nih.gov/pubmed/19419322.

314   Cordain, *Paleo Diet*, 112.

Dr. Cordain admits that alcohol consumption didn't precede agriculture and was not part of the diet of prehistoric humans. As such, the benefits of wine defy the theory that humankind genetically adapted to function best according to the diet that it evolved on over millions of years. Why single out wine to be included in the diet over other beneficial agricultural items such as legumes?

4. Why rule out sweet potatoes? Sweet potatoes are a great source of vitamin A, which studies show helps reduce the number of fat cells.[315] They have a healthy amount of numerous vitamins and minerals (including potassium, which Dr. Cordain recommends increasing). While they are high in carbohydrates, there are times when it is advantageous to increase carbohydrates. They are also sweet and filling, and have a low GI. I recommend them in moderation during a weight *maintenance* phase, so long as one's total carbohydrates remain at target level.

5. The evolutionary assumptions of Dr. Cordain's theories are disputed. Dr. Cordain writes, "The principles I have laid out in the Paleo Diet—all based on decades of scientific research and *proved over millions of years* by our ancestors—will make *your metabolism soar, your appetite shrink, and extra pounds begin to melt away* as you include more and more lean protein in your meals."[316]

Many scholars, doctors, professors, and scientists have written books disputing the theory of evolution with a variety of arguments and proofs. Since this is not the place to quote them all, I will suffice with a quote from Darwin himself:

There are, it must be admitted, cases of special difficulty opposed to the theory of natural selection...On this

---

315 S. M. Jeyakumar et al., "Vitamin A Supplementation Induces Adipose Tissue Loss through Apoptosis in Lean but Not in Obese Rats of the WNIN/OB Strain," *Journal of Molecular Endocrinology* (October 1, 2005), http://jme.endocrinology-journals.org/content/35/2/391.full.

316 Cordain, *The Paleo Diet*, 21.

doctrine of the extermination of an infinitude of connecting links, between the living and extinct inhabitants of the world, and at each successive period between the extinct and the still older species, why is not every geological formation charged with such links? Why does not every collection of fossil remains, afford plain evidence of the graduation and mutation of the forms of life… This is the most obvious of the many objections which may be urged against it…I can answer these questions and objections only on the supposition that the geological record is far more imperfect than most geologists believe.[317]

Over a century later, after much more fossil evidence has been uncovered, Stephen Jay Gould, professor of evolution at Harvard and perhaps the most respected and renowned proponent of the theory of evolution in our time, admits in his book *The Panda's Thumb*,

But if evolution proceeded as a lock step (in graduation), then the fossil record should display a pattern of gradual and sequential advance in organization. It does not, and I regard this failure as the most telling argument against an evolutionary ratchet…The extreme rarity of transitional forms in the fossil record persists as the trade secret of paleontology. The evolutionary trees that adorn our textbooks have data at the tips and nodes of their branches; the rest is inference…not the evidence of fossils.[318]

317 Charles Darwin, *The Origin of Species by Means of Natural Selection, or the Preservation of Favoured Races in the Struggle for Life*, London: John Murray, 6th edition (1876), 404–408.
318 Gould, *The Panda's Thumb*, 139.

THE VENICE NUTRITION PROGRAM
Body Confidence, *by Mark Macdonald*

Venice Nutrition comprises more than 350 consulting centers, four thousand nutrition "coaches," and 250,000 clients. This is an astounding accomplishment considering Macdonald (like myself) has no medical or dietetic licensing.

The Venice Nutrition Program is geared toward stabilizing blood sugar via three main principles:

1. A balanced meal should be eaten every three to four hours (five to six meals per day).
2. A nutrient ratio of 40 percent protein to 35 percent carbohydrates to 25 percent fat should be maintained.
3. The right amount of calories per meal should be identified and consumed.

Macdonald's book includes three secondary principles as well:

1. A meal should be eaten within an hour of waking.
2. A meal should be eaten within an hour of going to sleep.
3. When doing more than thirty-five minutes of high-intensity cardio training, people should include the consumption of protein during the activity.

Macdonald's guiding belief is that stable blood sugar is the key to losing fat. That is why he recommends constant meals throughout the day and restricting oneself to a modest amount of carbohydrates. In his words, "When the body's sugar is stable, it will continually release stored fat, which is then burned primarily within the muscle tissue through daily activity and exercise."[319]

---

319 Mark Macdonald, *Body Confidence*, (HarperCollins, 2011), 22.

Pros of the Venice Nutrition Program

1. Unlike the extreme low-carbohydrate approach of Atkins, which allows a mere 10 percent of caloric intake in the final maintenance stage, and unlike the extreme high-carbohydrate approach of the US Department of Health's recommendations of between 45 percent and 65 percent of caloric intake, the Venice recommendation of 35 percent is a moderately restricted-carbohydrate diet that helps stabilize blood sugar levels in a manner that you can feel comfortable with on a long-term basis.

2. Relative to most diets, this diet is low carbohydrate and high protein, which helps stabilize blood sugar levels, enables the continued burning of fat, reduces appetite and total caloric intake, and maintains muscle.

Cons of the Venice Nutrition Program

1. Eating a meal within an hour of waking is the opposite of what is recommended by the Talmud. It upsets the blood sugar balance, as explained in detail in chapter 7, because the hormone cortisol is at its daily peak half an hour after waking; therefore, eating a meal at that time spikes sugar levels up out of control. This causes hyperinsulinemia and adds unnecessary and unwanted calories.

2. Eating a meal within an hour of going to sleep is the opposite of what Maimonides recommends—three to four hours between mealtime and bedtime. Chapter 5 explains how eating shortly before bedtime worsens insulin resistance and hyperinsulinemia, impedes healthy digestion (thereby weakening the body), disrupts sleep, inhibits the release of the beneficial hormone HGH, impedes the beneficial effects of HGH, reduces the cleansing benefits of the nightly fast, and adds unnecessary and unwanted calories.

3. No advice is provided for the reduction of number of fat cells or improving leptin sensitivity, which are necessary for long-term fat reduction.

Criticism of the Venice Nutrition Program

Macdonald is a great fitness model, a justifiable reason to want to emulate him, making it understandable why so many people seek his advice. Some of his advice is surely good, but certain claims are misinformed. For example, Macdonald writes (pg. 118), "Since alcohol is void of nutrients, your body still needs to get its fuel somehow. That means if you drink alcohol without eating, your body will need to consume itself (primarily muscle) to provide the necessary fuel." In truth, alcohol has seven calories per gram—that's almost double the fuel of carbohydrates and proteins.

Another unsubstantiated claim is his attempt to "debunk the myth that doing cardio on an empty stomach burns fat."[320] He is correct that extended cardio on an empty stomach will also consume muscle; however, the process of gluconeogenesis burns protein and fat simultaneously, and so as long as the cardio is not overextended, only surplus proteins are consumed and not the actual muscle tissue. But in either case (moderate cardio or extended cardio), fats are burned when cardio is done on an empty stomach and obviously more so than after eating.

Macdonald's "debunking" is debunked by Professor Katarina T. Borer: "The limitation in the size of carbohydrate stores leads to metabolism of lipids during times of energy shortage."[321]

In other words, since carbohydrate stores will be lower on an empty stomach than on a full stomach, the body will be forced to fuel the exercise by burning *more* fat.

---

320 Ibid, 279.
321 Katarina T. Borer, *Advanced Exercise Endocrinology*, Human Kinetics (2013), 106.

THE DUKAN DIET
Dr. Pierre Dukan

Similar to Atkins, Dukan promotes a very low-carbohydrate diet. And as with Atkins, there are four phases: induction, ongoing weight loss, premaintenance, and lifetime maintenance (though Dukan gives different names to these phases). And like Atkins, his diet is so popular that it is impossible to ignore it or consider it a mere "fad." For our purposes, we need to highlight what is new and different about Dukan.

Phase 1: Induction (attack)
The average length is five days and zero caloric carbs. Unlike Atkins, Dukan severely restricts fats and includes 1.5 tablespoons of oat bran fiber. Dr. Dukan also stresses the importance of drinking enough water (at least 1.5 liters per day).

Phase 2: Ongoing weight loss (cruise)
The average length is two to six months. Oat bran fiber is increased to two tablespoons daily. Nonstarchy vegetables are added, alternating between a day of unrestricted (nonstarchy) vegetables and a day of only protein (like during the attack phase), with zero carbohydrates (no veggies).

Phase 3: Premaintenance (consolidation)
The length is five days for every pound lost (a person who lost twenty pounds in the first two phases will do this phase for one hundred days). Oat bran fiber remains at two tablespoons. The attack/pure-protein diet is reduced to only one day per week (Thursdays) instead of every other day. Two slices of whole wheat bread, one piece of fruit, and one portion of cheese are allowed each day. Two portions of starchy food (grains, legumes, or potatoes) are allowed per week. During the first half of the consolidation period (five days for every pound lost), you

may have one unrestricted meal per week—eating any food you desire, without overeating. And during the second half, you may have two "celebratory" meals per week.

Phase 4: Lifetime maintenance (stabilization)

The length is continual. Oat bran fiber is increased to three tablespoons. Six out of seven days are "unrestricted," while keeping to the good habits you have acquired, with one day per week of attack/ pure-protein diet (Thursdays). Take the stairs (not the elevator). In all the phases, Dukan stresses the importance of daily exercise. During the first two phases, keep the exercises light, such as walking, because the diet itself is very taxing. Afterward, more intense exercise is appropriate.

Pros of the Dukan Diet

1. This diet works quickly. The Dukan attack phase is the fastest way to lose fat while maintaining muscle. It is faster than Atkins because instead of burning ingested fats, the body is forced to burn stored body fat for energy.

2. This diet includes sufficient fiber. One of my biggest complaints with Atkins is the lack of fiber. Dukan solves that by stressing the importance of including a couple of tablespoons of oat bran fiber.

3. This diet is balanced and feasible. Unlike the Atkins maintenance phase that keeps carbohydrates below 10 percent, with Dukan, dieters are not so restrained for six days of the week. For many people this makes the difference between the impossible and the possible. The idea of permanently having one day per week of restricted carbohydrates is genius because it reduces one's glycogen reserves, ensuring insulin sensitivity and keeping you from storing fat as long as those reserves don't get filled up. (Extreme restriction from fats on that day, I think, is unnecessary.)

Cons of the Dukan Diet

1. For people who are capable of getting sufficient fiber in real food, that approach is preferred to supplementation because it allows consumption of the many micronutrients and bio-active compounds contained in high-fiber foods. Calories from vegetables slow down the short-term fat loss, but their benefits pay off in the long run, as vitamins A and D (plus calcium) help reduce fat cell numbers and improve leptin balance.
2. Phase 2 is quite difficult to adhere to. Many people might need a milder or slower approach.
3. Legumes are very healthy and high in fiber, protein, vitamins, and minerals. To totally abstain from them in phase 2 and re-strict them in phase 3 to two portions per week is too restrictive, in my opinion.
4. As with all diets, Dukan fails to address the problem that fat-mass decrease leads to a decrease in leptin. Without a way to increase leptin and improve leptin sensitivity, long term fat loss is very limited for most people.

Additional Comments

A person who carefully follows the Dukan instructions in the first two phases can expect dramatic short-term results. Most people desire a fast solution to obesity, and as Dukan delivers on this better than any other diet, it is no wonder he sold twenty million copies, and his book quickly became the most popular diet book of all time.

Dr. Dukan is of the opinion that most people want (and succeed better with) detailed diet instructions and a rigid plan, as opposed to being taught principles of physiology that enable each person to make adjustments for their personal circumstances. In contrast, the approach of *Maimonides and Metabolism* is to equip you with a deeper understand-ing of your physiology and how your hormones work so that you will know how to adapt your diet to any situation.

Dr. Dukan admits that many people who attempt his methods "manage to keep going for a while but then lose their way, and some of the weight they lost goes back on."[322] He also recognizes that with many people, "Resistance sets in, weight loss slows down, and one day the body resists a little more than on other days and weight loss comes to a halt."[323] Dukan's solution is as follows: "I prescribe what I call a 'blitz operation'…four days of the Attack diet's pure proteins without any deviation, restricting salt, etc.…."[324] This solution reminds me of how we used to fix the TV when we were kids. We'd smack it. If that didn't work, we'd smack it again. If necessary, we'd smack it harder. Heck, sometimes it worked!

It's safer to go with a more conservative approach. Even though the idea of *fast* weight loss is appealing, too often it sets up a fast rebound. Like charging into a slingshot, the faster one hits it, the faster one bounces in the opposite direction. That's another reason to include high-fiber vegetables in the first phases every day. Once the body is accustomed to Dukan's pure-protein attack, adding in necessary foods, such as vegetables, may be used by the body to halt fat loss.

Criticisms of the Dukan Diet

1. Dr. Dukan's advice is lipid-phobic. He writes, "Lipids (fats) are the absolute enemy of anyone trying to be slim…Since Atkins appeared, opening the way for lipids by demonizing carbohydrates…cholesterol and triglyceride levels rise dangerously, some people paying for this with their lives."[325]

    Refer to the studies in the previous chapter, most particularly the first study, and you will see that Dr. Dukan is wrong: cholesterol and triglyceride levels drop significantly on the

322 Pierre Dukan, *The Dukan Diet* (Hodder and Stoughton, 2010), 268.
323 Ibid, 290.
324 Ibid, 291.
325 Ibid, 18.

Atkins very low-carbohydrate diet, despite the dieter ingesting more lipids.

See also the meta-analyses at the end of the previous chapter, particularly the second one. Very low-carbohydrate diets that are fueled primarily by proteins and lipids help lower insulin and glucose levels, a very important benefit for diabetics and prediabetics.

Omega-3 is an essential fat required to include in the diet, and certain vitamins require dietary fats to be absorbed. Reducing dietary fats to a minimum helps speed fat loss, but there's no reason to go overboard by creating a fear of one of the three macronutrients.

There's another advantage to fats over proteins; fats fill you up without any insulin response, while proteins induce an insulin response, and insulin blocks the body's breakdown of stored body fat.

2. There is a fat cell number blooper in the book that is misleading. Healthy adults have between twenty-five and thirty billion fat cells, which contain about twenty to twenty-five pounds of fat. When fat mass increases, the fat cells stretch like balloons to contain it. The average size (weight) of an adult fat cell is about 0.6 micrograms, but they can vary in size from 0.2 micrograms to 0.9 micrograms.

When a person puts on fat, at first that stretches the fat cells without changing the number, but as time goes by, if the added fat mass remains, the body adapts by gradually adding more fat cells. That explains why a typical person who has been overweight for years can have fifty to seventy-five billion fat cells to accommodate their twenty to sixty excess pounds of fat (beyond the twenty to twenty-five pounds of healthy fat mass).

The way *The Dukan Diet* explains fat cell increase leads to a seriously mistaken perception: that a person can put on fat up to a 28 BMI without adding fat cells, and if they continue to put on more fat, somewhere between 28 and 29 BMI, their twenty-five billion fat cells suddenly all simultaneously divide in two, yielding a total of fifty billion fat cells instantaneously! Dr. Dukan writes,[326]

> It is important to pinpoint simply and concretely the moment in their weight history when there is this risk of cell division...If the weight gain continues, the adipocytes hypertrophy, or enlarge, and reach the limit of their elasticity. At this critical moment, any additional weight gain triggers a new and exceptional event, completely changing the future and prognosis for weight problems. No longer able to contain any more fat the adipocyte cell DIVIDES into two daughter adipocyte cells. This simple division suddenly doubles the body's capacity to make and store fat...I was able to work out statistics that enabled me to pinpoint this moment as being after BMI 28 has been reached and going toward BMI 29.

3. The Dukan diet oversimplifies the time needed to adapt to new lower body weight. Dr. Dukan writes,[327] "The high-risk period for regaining weight lasts about five days for every pound lost, 30 days or a month for six to seven pounds, and 100 days for a loss of 18–20 pounds."

There are more factors that influence the length of the high-risk period, such as how long the person was overweight. If a person recently put on twenty pounds, the time period in which there is a high risk of regaining the lost weight (once they've gotten rid of it) is short compared to a person who has been living for many

---

326 Dukan, *The Dukan Diet*, 227–28.
327 Ibid, 109.

years with the extra twenty pounds, as his or her body has accustomed itself to the higher weight with a corresponding number of fat cells. The person who has been overweight for years has a higher homeostatic weight level, which their body is naturally set to.

Another influencing factor is the percentage of fat mass lost. For a 130-pound woman who dropped weight to 110, the loss of twenty pounds of fat (i.e., 50 percent of her total fat mass) will take much longer to acclimate to than a six-hundred-pound obese man, whose twenty-pound loss constitutes less than a mere 5 percent of his total fat mass. This woman will have a dramatic reduction in circulating leptin, as her fat mass has been cut in half. This man won't experience a significant reduction in leptin, because his fat mass only decreased by 5 percent.

4. Some of Dr. Dukan's recommendations are desperate and dangerous. Dr. Dukan recommends taking cold showers, sucking on ice cubes, and eating one's food cold.[328] These methods will burn calories, but there is a risk of becoming ill. Losing fat reduces leptin, which weakens the immune system. Combining extreme dieting with cold showers may push people beyond their limits.

---

328 Ibid, 229-33.

THE SOUTH BEACH DIET
Dr. Arthur Agatston

The South Beach diet recommends three meals and two snacks per day and has three phases.

Phase 1: Two weeks—moderately fast fat loss
The main purpose of this phase is to stabilize blood sugar and eliminate cravings. The main restriction in this phase is complete abstinence from starchy foods (grains, potatoes, etc.) and sugar. No fruits or high-calorie vegetables are allowed. Meat and dairy are restricted to lean cuts of meat and low-fat dairy.

Phase 2: Two weeks (or longer)—transition phase
This phase reintroduces healthy carbohydrates into the diet, which were completely restricted in phase 1. Healthy carbohydrates are whole grains and fresh fruits (high fiber plus a low glycemic index) as opposed to refined grains, processed junk food, beets, corn, white potatoes, canned and dried fruit, honey, sugar, or jelly. This phase begins by adding one portion per day of healthy carbohydrates plus one piece of fruit per day and gradually raises carbohydrate intake to three portions per day plus three pieces of fruit.

Phase 3: Continuous lifestyle
This phase continues where phase 2 left off with the addition of "occasional sinful treats." In all phases, trans fats are off-limits, and saturated fats are minimized.

Pros of the South Beach Diet
1. This very simple and conservative approach is easy to follow and does not upset one's equilibrium. Other more aggressive weight-loss methods lead to the yo-yo effect of fast weight loss followed by the inevitable rebound.

2. The book has educational value, teaching important basics of diet and exercise.

Cons of the South Beach Diet

1. This diet is not potent enough to take off stubborn pounds or to take off many pounds for those who are severely overweight. This is essentially a list of healthy foods to eat and unhealthy foods to avoid. For people struggling with obesity, this is insufficient. It merely qualifies as advice for weight maintenance, as opposed to fat-loss strategies.
2. No advice is provided for reduction of the number of fat cells or improving leptin sensitivity, both of which are necessary for long-term fat reduction.

THE ZONE DIET
Dr. Barry Sears

Whereas the Zone diet shares the common goal of conquering obesity, unlike other diets that take direct approaches to weight loss, Zone's direct focus first and foremost is on achieving the hormonal balance that will rectify the root problem of the metabolic syndrome—hyperinsulinemia. Without the adverse effects of hyperinsulinemia, one's body weight normalizes naturally on its own.

1. **Macronutrient division.** Each of the three daily meals and two snacks should have a macronutrient caloric division of 40 percent carbohydrates, 30 percent protein, and 30 percent fat.
2. **Plan total daily caloric intake.** Calculate your daily grams of required protein: your lean body mass in pounds, multiplied by activity factor. Activity factor is between 0.5 and 1.0:
   - Sedentary: 0.5
   - Light exercise (walking): 0.6
   - Moderate (ninety minutes per week): 0.7
   - Active (five hours per week): 0.8
   - Very active (ten hours per week): 0.9
   - Heavy weight training (five times per week): 1.0

   To calculate lean body mass, subtract body fat from total weight. For example, a 154-pound *sedentary* male with thirty-six pounds of fat has a lean body mass of 118 pounds. Multiplied by the factor 0.5, this results in a daily requirement of fifty-nine grams of protein. Divide daily protein into eleven parts. Breakfast, lunch, and dinner make up three parts each (nine total), with one part late-afternoon snack and one part late-night snack.
3. **Never skip a meal or snack.** You should never go more than five hours between meals or snacks. Plan to start with an early

breakfast, lunch within five hours of breakfast, an afternoon snack, dinner, and a late-night snack before bed. By avoiding long breaks from eating, you keep blood sugar levels from dropping.

4. **Choose healthy food sources.** That includes low-fat protein sources, high-fiber carbohydrate sources, and monounsaturated fats preferred to alternative fats.

5. **Avoid eating more than five hundred calories per meal.** If your requirements are very high (NFL players), eat more than three full meals per day.

6. **Get sufficient EPA (omega-3).** This comes either from fish or supplements.

7. **Eat three to five portions of cooked oatmeal per week.** The fiber in oatmeal is particularly beneficial for heart health. Oatmeal contains both calcium and potassium, critical nutrients that are insufficient in the typical diet.

Pros of the Zone Diet

1. Compared to the typical high-carbohydrate diet (55 to 65 percent), the Zone diet reduces hyperinsulinemia and improves hormonal and blood sugar stability.

2. It reduces hunger due to a higher than typical protein intake and due to the stabilizing of blood sugar levels.

3. It lowers triglycerides and serum cholesterol by stabilizing blood sugar levels.

4. Since this diet has no fast-fat-loss phase, there are no "rebounds."

5. The diet is easy to adhere to. It is completely natural, without the stress of food-category restrictions.

Cons of the Zone Diet

1. Dr. Sears recommends late-night snacks to prevent sugar levels from dropping too low if one goes without food for too long. However, this logic ignores the fact that cortisol begins

to rise just a couple hours after going to bed, maintaining sugar levels by burning fat. The unnecessary late-night snack prevents the burning of fat. Late-night snacks also cause digestive problems,[329, 330] raise blood pressure thereby disturbing rest,[331] inhibit the release of HGH,[332, 333] stifle the effectiveness of whatever HGH is released,[334] and minimize the benefits of daily intermittent fasting, as discussed in chapters 5 and 9.

2. An early breakfast is counterproductive, as explained at length in chapter 7. There is no reason to fear that blood sugar levels will drop in the early morning on an empty stomach because cortisol is at its daily peak half an hour after waking. Having a full sized breakfast that consists of 40 percent carbohydrates is terrible if the breakfast is early, because when cortisol levels are high, the body is resistant to insulin, forcing the body to release high doses of insulin to lower blood sugar, which later leads to sugar lows.

3. For many overweight people, the lower carbohydrates and increased protein of this diet make them healthier and stabilize their weight, but they do not lose significant amounts of weight.

329 R.O Dantas and C. G. Aben-Athar, "Aspects of Sleep Effects on the Digestive Tract," *Arquivos de gastroenterologia* 1 (January–March 2002): 55–9. http://www.ncbi.nlm.nih.gov/pubmed/12184167.

330 Hye-kyung Jung, Rok Seon Choung, and Nicholas J. Talley, "Gastroesophageal Reflux Disease and Sleep Disorders: Evidence for a Causal Link and Therapeutic Implications," *Journal of Neurogastroenterology and Motility* (January 2010), http://www.ncbi.nlm.nih.gov/pmc/articles/PMC2879818/.

331 Ibid.

332 R. Lanzi et al., "Elevated Insulin Levels Contribute to the Reduced Growth Hormone (GH) Response to GH-Releasing Hormone in Obese Subjects," *Metabolism* (1999), http://www.ncbi.nlm.nih.gov/pubmed/10484056.

333 Hiroo Imura et al., "Effect of Adrenergic-Blocking or -Stimulating Agents on Plasma Growth Hormone, Immunoreactive Insulin, and Blood Free Fatty Acid Levels in Man," *Journal of Clinical Investigation* 50, no. 5 (May 1971), http://www.jci.org/articles/view/106578.

334 Shaonin Ji et al., "Insulin Inhibits Growth Hormone **Signaling via the Growth Hormone Receptor/JAK2/STAT5B Pathway**," *Journal of Biological Chemistry* (May 7, 1999), http://www.jbc.org/content/274/19/13434.full.

4. No advice is provided for reduction of the number of fat cells or for improving leptin sensitivity, which is necessary for long-term fat reduction.

Notes

The book is very educational, and all the advice is good (except for late-night snacks and early breakfasting).

Dr. Sears insists that each meal and snack rigidly maintain the caloric proportions of 40 percent carbohydrates, 30 percent protein, and 30 percent fat. Since a primary focus of the Zone diet is to reverse hyperinsulinemia, I question his insistence on always combining carbohydrates with proteins, as numerous studies have shown that the addition of proteins to a portion of carbohydrates *increases* the insulin response despite lowering glucose levels.[335, 336]

335   Luc J. C. van Loon et al., "Amino Acid Ingestion Strongly Enhances Insulin Secretion in Patients With Long-Term Type 2 Diabetes," *Diabetes Care* (2003), http://care.diabetes-journals.org/content/26/3/625.full.
336   Frank Q Nuttall et al., "Effect of Protein Ingestion on the Glucose and Insulin Response to a Standardized Oral Glucose Load," Diabetes Care (1984), http://care.diabetesjournals.org/content/26/3/625.full.

THE FAST DIET
Dr. Michael Mosley and Mimi Spencer

The Fast Diet attempts to utilize the metabolic and weight-loss benefits of intermittent fasting. Their recommendations include the following:

1. "Fasting" two nonconsecutive days per week. The "fast" day includes five hundred calories for women and six hundred for men, divided between two meals that are twelve hours apart, such as 7:30 a.m. and 7:30 p.m. Alternatives to this plan are either dividing the five hundred or six hundred calories between two meals and an additional two light snacks or limiting the entire caloric intake to one meal.
2. The five or six hundred calories of the fast day should be high in lean protein (fifty grams equaling two hundred calories) and include low-glycemic carbohydrates.
3. In the optimal maintenance model, one can fast twice a week continuously, or reduce to only one fast per week. When in need of weight reduction, one can always revert temporarily to having two (or even three) fasts per week.

Pros of the Fast Diet
1. Two days a week of extreme calorie restriction helps reduce body fat in most people *in the short term*.
2. The fast days greatly reduce glycogen reserves, improving insulin sensitivity in the days following the fast.

Cons of the Fast Diet
1. Breakfast at 7:30 a.m. is too early, as cortisol is at its peak then. This causes insulin resistance, drives up sugar levels too early in the day, and rebounds with a sugar low, making it difficult to avoid eating before 7:30 p.m.

2. Skipping meals will wreak havoc by increasing ghrelin.[337] Ghrelin increases hunger and directs metabolism to store fat (as opposed to burning it) and induces secretion of gastric acid and pancreatic enzymes, thereby increasing energy absorption (extracting calories more efficiently, such that the body absorbs what it needs for maintaining body weight).[338] Doing this twice a week over a period of time is *likely to increase the number of fat cells*,[339] thereby resetting one's fat-homeostasis level to a heavier weight. Leptin levels fall, and inevitably the dieter gains back all he or she has lost—and more.

3. When consuming only five or six hundred calories in a day, the body consumes its own muscle to compensate for the caloric deficit such that most of the lost weight is not fat. If nearly all the ingested calories were protein (as the Dukan diet recommends), this problem could be avoided, but Dr. Mosley recommends including only fifty grams of protein during "fast" days.

Criticisms of the Fast Diet

Dr. Mosley is a licensed medical doctor, but instead of pursuing a career practicing medicine, he became (in his own words, from the flap of his book) a "science journalist, producer, and TV personality." Mimi Spencer (coauthor of *The Fast Diet*) is a journalist and author. It appears that the television and journalistic promotion of this diet made it popular more so than any benefits of following the diet.

---

337   H. S. Callahan et al., "Postprandial Suppression of Plasma Ghrelin Level Is Proportional to Ingested Caloric Load but Does Not Predict Intermeal Interval in Humans," *Journal of Clinical Endocrinology and Metabolism* (March 2004), http://www.ncbi.nlm.nih.gov/pubmed/15001628.

338   Chih-Yen Chen et al., "Ghrelin Gene Products and the Regulation of Food Intake and Gut Motility," *Pharmacological Reviews* (December 2009), http://pharmrev.aspetjournals.org/content/61/4/430.full#ref-91.

339   M. S. Kim et al., "The Mitogenic and Antiapoptotic Actions of Ghrelin in 3t3-L1 Adipocytes," Molecular endocrinology (Baltimore, Md.) (September 2004), http://www.ncbi.nlm.nih.gov/pubmed/15178745.

Dr. Mosley bases his recommendations on numerous studies that show the benefits of intermittent fasting. But I found no precedent for this method, nor any studies that demonstrate the long-term effects of his particular application of intermittent "fasting." In *The No-Fad Diet*,[340] The American Heart Association warns against skipping meals, the dangers of which were explained just above.

---

340 American Heart Association, *The No-Fad Diet* (2011), Introduction, X.

THE NO-FAD DIET
American Heart Association

The AHA claims that fad diets may work temporarily but do not lead to permanent weight loss. They write, "Signs of an unhealthy or fad diet include: a drastic reduction in calories without regard for adequate nutrition; a dependence on powders, herbs, or pills; a reliance on certain foods or food combinations; an elimination of carbs, fat, or any other type of food; a recommendation to skip meals or replace meals with drinks or food bars."

1. For weight loss, you should strive for a deficit of five hundred calories per day to lose one pound per week, or a deficit of one thousand calories per day to lose two pounds per week. Choose between or combine the following three strategies of calorie reduction:
   b. Substitute high-calorie foods with lower calorie foods. For example, instead of having a glass of orange juice, eat an orange. Instead of having a regular soft drink, substitute it with a sugar-free one. Instead of eating regular cheddar cheese, go for the low-fat version.
   c. Reduce portion size.
   d. Try the American Heart Association's menu plans.
2. The diet should be rich in nutrient-dense foods from these major food groups: vegetables and fruits; whole grains; low-fat dairy; fish; lean cuts of meat and poultry; legumes, nuts, and seeds; and unsaturated oils and fats.
3. Avoid trans fats, and limit cholesterol to less than three hundred milligrams per day (recently the AHA has nullified its restriction on dietary cholesterol).
4. Limit salt to less than fifteen hundred milligrams per day.
5. Limit added sugars to less than 150 calories per day for men and one hundred calories per day for women.

6. Limit alcoholic beverages to no more than two per day for men and one per day for women.
7. If you're not hungry, don't eat.
8. Keep snacks low in calories.
9. Begin meals with a zero-calorie drink or a low-calorie starter.

Pros of the No-Fad Diet
1. Avoiding excess salt, sugar, and trans fats and eating varied and balanced, nutrient-dense food is solid, time-tested advice.
2. Beginning a meal with a zero-calorie drink helps you feel sated by fewer calories.
3. Cutting calories helps some people lose weight, at least in the short term.

Cons of the No-Fad Diet
1. As explained at length in part I, calorie-restricted diets usually increase ghrelin, which can lead to an increased number of fat cells, reduce leptin, and set one's homeostatic fat-mass level to a heavier level, leading to weight gain.
2. No advice is provided for reducing the number of fat cells or improving leptin sensitivity, which are necessary for long-term fat reduction.

Criticisms of the No-Fad Diet
1. **Not all calories were created equal.** The previous chapter included many studies and meta-analyses demonstrating the clear advantages of low-carbohydrate, high-protein diets for weight loss and other parameters (such as sugar stability, lowered triglycerides, etc.). In fact it is undisputed that low-carbohydrate diets are especially advantageous for short-term weight loss. These studies span decades and are well known. Yet the American Heart Association claims that "a calorie is a calorie

no matter what the macronutrient source is."[341] They base this claim on a single study (for which they do not provide any details—date, authors, or name of study), writing, "In a recent study from the National Institutes of Health, experts compared four different diets representing a range of percentages of fat, protein, and carbohydrates, and they found that all subjects lost about the same amount of weight."[342]

The only study I am aware of that compares four different diets is a twelve-month study published in the *Journal of the American Medical Association*, in 2007.[343] In it, 311 women were randomly assigned to follow the Atkins (very low carbohydrate), Zone (moderate to low carbohydrate), LEARN (high carbohydrate, low fat, based on national guidelines), or Ornish (very high carbohydrate) diets for twelve months. The study concludes, "The Atkins group on average lost roughly double the weight each of the other groups, and experienced more favorable overall metabolic effects at 12 months (4.7 kg—10.3 lb.). Weight loss was not statistically different among the Zone, LEARN, and Ornish groups. Zone (1.6 kg—3.5 lb.), LEARN (2.6 kg—5.7 lb.), and Ornish (2.2 kg—4.9 lb.)."

I am surprised that the American Heart Association published this diet book in 2005 and again in 2011, writing the above (that all types of divisions of macronutrients lead to the same weight loss), when in 2003, a six-month study *that was sponsored by the American Heart Association* was published in the *Journal of*

---

341   American Heart Association, *The No-Fad Diet* (2011), 13.

342   Ibid, 13.

343   Christopher D. Gardner et al., "Comparison of the Atkins, Zone, Ornish, and Learn Diets for Change in Weight and Related Risk Factors among Overweight Premenopausal Women: The A to Z Weight Loss Study," *Journal of the American Medical Association* (2007), http://jama.jamanetwork.com/article.aspx?articleid=205916.

Clinical Endocrinology and Metabolism,[344] comparing the effects of a very low-carbohydrate (Atkins) diet to a low-fat diet conforming to the guidelines currently recommended by the American Heart Association, concluding that the "very-low-carb (Atkins) diet is more than doubly effective than the American Heart Association's low-fat diet for short-term weight loss (−18.7 lb. vs. −8.6 lb.)."

2. **The calorie deficit myth.** The AHA promotes the idea that weight loss is pure and simple mathematics. They write,[345] "A calorie is a calorie. To create weight loss, you must change the balance in favor of calories out...Subtract about 500 calories per day to lose about 1 pound per week. Subtract about 1,000 calories per day to lose about 2 pounds per week."

The calculation is based on the fact that a pound of fat is 3,500 calories; therefore, a deficit of five hundred calories multiplied by seven days per week equals 3,500 calories, which is equal to one pound of fat.

But this ignores the fact that calorie restriction quickly leads to a slower metabolism and more effective digestion that extracts more calories per portion.[346] They themselves admit,[347] "Most people experience a decrease in metabolism at middle-age," demonstrating their awareness that a person's changing metabolism makes calorie calculating a complex issue. So why do they mislead people with their simplified math of "a calorie is a calorie" and ignore the fact that calorie restriction also slows metabolism?

---

344 Bonnie J. Brehm et al., "A Randomized Trial Comparing a Very Low Carbohydrate Diet and a Calorie-Restricted Low Fat Diet on Body Weight and Cardiovascular Risk Factors in Healthy Women," *Journal of Clinical Endocrinology & Metabolism* (2003), http://press.endocrine.org/doi/full/10.1210/jc.2002-021480.

345 American Heart Association, *The No-Fad Diet* (2011), 12-13.

346 Chih-Yen Chen et al., "Ghrelin Gene Products and the Regulation of Food Intake and Gut Motility," *Pharmacological Reviews* (December 2009), http://pharmrev.aspetjournals.org/content/61/4/430.full#ref-91.

347 American Heart Association, *The No-Fad Diet* (2011), 16.

In part I, I explained why this misinformation is harmful, leading some people to gain weight and leading dieters to think they are at fault for gaining back the lost weight. But to briefly recap, restricting calories increases ghrelin, which when chronic, leads to an increased number of fat cells, lower leptin levels, and an increase in the homeostatic fat-mass level.

16

Combining the Most Effective Methods for Short-Term and Long-Term Fat Loss

This chapter puts all the pieces of the puzzle together. Part II, chapters 4 through 9 explained in detail the four primary elements of combating the metabolic syndrome. Part III, chapters 7 through 10 delved into the macronutrients, explaining what and how much protein to include in your diet, the importance of low carbohydrates yet high fiber, and what foods supply high fiber, what fats to avoid, and what fats to increase for overall health. In part IV, we explored many studies demonstrating the clear advantages of maintaining a low-carbohydrate diet, at least during phases of weight loss, and we examined a variety of dieting techniques. All this comes together in this final chapter, primarily in implementing *permanent diet and exercise policies*, as well as occasionally incorporating a *temporary high-speed fat-loss plan*, explaining how and when to transition between these two plans. This chapter includes the following:

- Permanent Diet and Exercise Policies
- Temporary High-Speed Fat-Loss Plan
- Transitional Phase from Fat-Loss to Permanent Policies
- When to Use the Temporary Fat-Loss Plan
- Fat-Loss Phase and Maintenance Phase—Why Both?

- How to Transition between Fat-Loss and Fat-Maintenance Plans
- The Physiology of the Very Low-Carbohydrate Diet
- Glycogen Reserve Capacity and Body-Weight Fluctuation
- Record Parameters before Changing Your Diet

Outlined below are the practical applications of the numerous nutritional details presented in earlier chapters. (For the physiology and endocrinology theory with supporting studies and sources, refer to previous chapters). By occasionally referring back to this summary you can keep yourself on track to improved health.

PERMANENT DIET AND EXERCISE POLICIES

1. Gradually adapt to an early dinnertime (little to no food three to four hours before sleep).
2. Incorporate daily aerobic exercise into your schedule before breakfast. At the very least, get your body warmed up with a couple of minutes of exertion (jumping jacks, running in place, and/or a few flights of stairs) before breakfast.
3. Gradually adapt to late breakfast (three to six hours after waking). A prebreakfast snack is recommended one and a half to two hours after waking.
4. Minimize nutrient-empty carbohydrates (sugar, refined grains, and potatoes).
5. Soak up sunlight regularly (or supplement with vitamin D).
6. Consume a high-protein and high-calcium diet that includes fish and high-protein, low-fat dairy. (Sardines, salmon, and dairy are high in calcium; fish also have the benefits of omega-3s.)
7. Eat a high-fiber diet (from food sources high in nutrients): a tablespoon of chia seed and ground flaxseed each day plus high-fiber vegetables—specifically vegetables high in vitamin A, such as carrots and sweet potatoes. You can also supplement with a few tablespoons of bran.

8. Perform resistance training (preferably in the late afternoon, but certainly not before breakfast) three times per week.

9. Make sure to get sufficient nutrients while minimizing salt and saturated fats. The In their 2015 report, the DGAC (Dietary Guidelines Advisory Committee) characterized these as short-fall nutrients: vitamin A, vitamin D, vitamin E, vitamin C, folate, calcium, magnesium, fiber, and potassium. Of the shortfall nutrients, calcium, vitamin D, fiber, and potassium also are classified as nutrients of public health concern because their underconsumption has been linked in the scientific literature to adverse health outcomes. Furthermore, the DGAC writes that the typical intake is too high for refined grains, added sugars, sodium, and saturated fat.

10. When eating meat and dairy products, opt for the grass-fed variety for the amazing benefits of CLA (conjugated linoleic acid). Grass-fed meat and dairy contains three to five times the amount of CLA than grain fattened, while containing significantly less saturated fats. See our website idealmetabolism.com to locate where to buy the best quality grass-fed meat and dairy products. See chapter 13 for details on the benefits of CLA.

TEMPORARY HIGH-SPEED FAT-LOSS PLAN

The fastest way to lose weight is to completely stop eating, but long-term fasting leads to a loss of muscle and a depletion of nutrients that the body depends on for health. In order to avoid these problems, you need to eat sufficient protein for protein homeostasis and include fiber and necessary micronutrients. Certain micronutrients are absorbed together with fats, others with carbohydrates, requiring at least a small amount of these macronutrients in the diet. This is a strict and difficult diet, but it is very effective and need only be used short term.

1. Adhere to a diet with an extreme reduction in carbohydrates: no bread, pasta, rice, or any other grain. No sugar. No potatoes.

Limit carbohydrates to high-fiber varieties (vegetables), including vegetables high in vitamin A.

2. Obtain sufficient amounts of omega-3s, but otherwise *minimize fat ingestion*. Certain vitamins are fat soluble; therefore, avoiding fats completely can lead to deficiencies. A teaspoon per day of coconut oil boosts metabolism and reduces appetite. Chia and flaxseed contain omega-3 plus fiber, vitamins, and minerals. Fats can suppress appetite and slow down digestion, keeping us full longer. But ingesting more fat than needed will block the burning of stored fat, which is our goal.

3. Since the body will be running on a high-caloric deficit, the RDA of protein—0.8 grams per kilogram of body weight—will not be nearly sufficient for protein homeostasis and maintenance of muscle mass. Once the supply of glycogen stored in the liver nears zero, the body begins to convert fats and proteins into glucose to fuel the brain and other organs that are glucose dependent. Some organs are capable of burning fat directly as fuel, and the muscles are also capable of burning three amino acids as fuel (known as branched-chain amino acids—BCAAs). The body also converts fats and *amino acids* into glucose in a process known as gluconeogenesis, burning a significant portion of protein as fuel.

The ideal level of protein intake would be the least amount that would maintain protein homeostasis. When one takes in less than that amount, the body consumes its own muscle for fuel. If one consumes more than that amount, one burns less fat. Since it's impossible to know exactly the ideal level, the practice is to be on the safe side and consume a bit extra, so as not to lose the hard-earned muscle, weaken the body, and lower one's basic metabolic rate. When the amino acid glutamine runs low due to being converted to glucose, the immune system can be compromised, risking illness. Having a little more protein than necessary only slightly slows down fat loss, because using protein as fuel is inefficient. Ingesting five hundred calories of protein more than necessary for protein homeostasis won't prevent you from burning off five hundred calories of fat, because many of those calories are lost when converted to glucose (as the conversion is inefficient). Also, "extra" amino acids are often "lost into the urine."[348] Certain amino acids can be converted to acetyl-CoA, which can then be synthesized into triglycerides (fat),[349] such that eating extraordinary amounts of protein, even without fat and carbohydrates, can theoretically lead to fat gain. But since the body has a natural repulsion to overeating protein, most people don't need to limit protein intake. By eating protein to satiety, you avoid increasing ghrelin.

4. Continue with the permanent diet policies, with the exception that resistance training should be with lighter weights and/or reduced workout times and frequencies. Also, the intensity of aerobic workouts should be reduced, but the duration can be maintained; aerobic workouts can even be extended if it won't be too stressful for one's fitness condition.

5. The length of the extreme-carbohydrate-reduction phase can be as little as one day or as long as excess fat mass continues to reduce without significant resistance (as long as six months or even a year, in extreme cases). Typically the extreme reduction phase would be two to four weeks, with a gradual transition back to the permanent phase over an additional span of two to four weeks. Since this plan is extremely effective in fat loss, it is important to coordinate the length and strictness of its use with a licensed dietitian or doctor to ensure that it is appropriate for the individual.

---

348   Guyton and Hall, *Textbook of Medical Physiology*, Saunders (2011), 833.
349   Ibid., 825.

TRANSITIONAL PHASE FROM FAT-LOSS TO PERMANENT POLICIES

Gradually reintroduce carbohydrates (whole grains and potatoes), while gradually returning to more intensive exercise and heavier weight lifting.

WHEN TO USE THE TEMPORARY FAT-LOSS PLAN

Anytime one's waistband is expanding is a time to switch to a temporary weight-loss mode. But late January is the best time of the year to start, according to Rabbi Klonimus Kalman Epstein.[350] One reason is to counterbalance the increased appetite at that time.[351] (Appetite increases with cold weather and also with the increasing length of daylight.[352] In early winter, daylight hours are shrinking, but in late January, it is both cold and a time of increasing daylight hours—increasing appetite.) Another consideration is that seasonal body weight is highest around January 18 and lowest around July 18,[353] making the end of January a good opportunity to catch a ride on the seasonal weight-loss wave. Additionally, it is best to get to one's seasonal lowest weight much earlier than July, in order to maximize the apoptosis benefits of the summer sun. *Vitamin D from the sun combined with calcium in the diet can help reduce the number of fat cells if fat mass is already significantly lower than one's personal accustomed weight.*

---

350   Rabbi Klonimus Kalman Epstein, "Remizai TuBiShvat," *Meor VaShemesh* (1822).
351   Ibid.
352   Clare L. Adam and Julian G. Mercer, "Appetite Regulation and Seasonality: Implications for Obesity," *Proceedings of the Nutrition Society* (2004), http://journals.cambridge.org/download.php?file=%2FPNS%2FPNS63_03%2FS0029665104000564a.pdf&code=6a678e2eed7163170244640216120c97.
353   Dawn Schwenke, "Seasonal Fluctuation in Weight is Not Associated with Weight Gain," *Circulation* (2010), http://circ.ahajournals.org/cgi/content/meeting_abstract/122/21_MeetingAbstracts/A21291.

FAT-LOSS PHASE AND MAINTENANCE
PHASE—WHY BOTH?

The following explains why a maintenance plan doesn't work for significant fat loss and why a fat loss plan doesn't work long-term.

As explained in chapter 1, fat mass is regulated by the hormone leptin to maintain status quo. In the long term, this hormone acts against changes (either up or down) in fat mass. The permanent plan in most cases will have very positive effects on health, especially insulin sensitivity. The permanent plan also makes fat-loss phases easier to handle and more effective because you are accustomed to longer hours of daily intermittent fasting and because of improved insulin sensitivity. And vitamin D increases leptin sensitivity, thereby reducing hunger.[354] However, since the permanent plan allows you to eat without caloric restriction, it works primarily for maintenance and only reduces body fat in some people mildly.

The fat-loss plan is inappropriate for long-term use because when fat mass goes down, so does the hormone leptin, slowing metabolism and enforcing a limit as to how much fat loss one's body will tolerate by increasing hunger. *Instead of fighting against one's body, it is usually more productive to transition from fat loss to weight maintenance until the body has adapted to the lower fat mass.* Then you can transition back to fat loss without resistance from the body. Compared to other diets, during the first six months, the very low-carbohydrate fat-loss plan has proven by far to be the fastest way to lose fat, but later its greater effectiveness diminishes. After a break from very low-carbohydrate dieting (switching to the maintenance plan), the effectiveness of the very low-carbohydrate diet can be regained. Attempting the intense short-term fat-loss plan for too long a period can have several negative effects:

1. Such a diet is stressful and weakens the immune system. If used intensely for too long, one can become ill.

354 Michael Holick, *The Vitamin D Solution* (Hudson Street Press, 2010), 16.

2. If one sets fat-loss goals that are too difficult, the frustration of not reaching those goals can lead to abandonment of the whole project. There comes a point when progress in fat loss diminishes to the point of not being worth the effort of sticking to the stressful very low-carbohydrate diet, so don't plan on pushing yourself into a no-win situation.

The fat-loss plan is also inappropriate for strength-building and muscle-building programs. Body builders conventionally alternate between muscle-building periods and fat-cutting periods, because during a fat-cutting period, the body cannot absorb enough protein and nutrition to recover in a timely fashion from the stresses of exercise. Insulin is needed to speed the muscle's uptake of nutrients, and insulin works in opposition of fat burning.

HOW TO TRANSITION BETWEEN FAT-LOSS AND FAT-MAINTENANCE PLANS

This was elaborated on in part I. The basic goal is to reduce fat mass to the lowest level that does *not* cause the body to fight the loss by slowing metabolism, extracting a greater percentage of ingested nutrients, and increasing hunger. The next step is to maintain the lowered fat-mass level until the body adapts by reducing fat cell numbers and becoming more sensitive to reduced leptin levels. Once adapted, you can return to another round of fat loss, followed by maintenance, etcetera.

The fat-loss phase is clear as outlined above. One strategy is to make the fat-loss phase work as fast as possible, to minimize the time under caloric-deficit stress, and maximize the time available for muscle building. When opting for this strategy, you minimize carbohydrates (and calories) as much as possible without harming health by failing to get enough protein, fiber, vitamins, and minerals. Be sure to eat protein to satiety to avoid inducing chronic hunger, which is harmful because it increases ghrelin.

The permanent phase is also clear as outlined above.

In the transition phase, the goal is to maintain the lowered fat-mass level until the body is so well adapted that there is no longer a tendency toward weight gain.

It would be nice if we could simply gradually add back into the diet healthy carbohydrates until we're back on the long-term plan with unrestricted calories. However, the unfortunate reality for many is that there is a tendency to edge upward on the scale when doing so.

Here are three alternatives to counter that tendency:

1. Remain on the fat-loss diet, but with a little leniency, allow-ing just a small amount of carbohydrates such that weight drifts neither up nor down. The drawbacks to this are that staying on a restricted diet long term is a strain, there is a danger of not being able to stick to the plan, and it is not at all appropriate to use this strategy simultaneously with training for increased muscle mass.

2. Ignore the scale for a few weeks. Live a normal, unrestricted life according to the long-term health policies above, and when reenergized for battle, return to the strict fat-loss program for a week or so. The drawback to this is that the hard earned fat-loss success will be sustained for too short a time to effectively reduce fat cell numbers.

3. Live the normal unrestricted life for five to six days per week, and on one or two days per week, go to nearly zero carbohy-drates. This can be very effective, yet for this to succeed, it is important to understand the physiology of the very low-carbo-hydrate diet, which will be explained shortly.

4. Combine strategies 1 and 3. Instead of five to six days of an unrestricted diet, make some days mildly restricted, with one or two days nearly carbohydrate-free.

THE BENEFIT OF ALTERNATING ONE'S DIET

Some dietitians recommend avoiding "crash-diets"; they propose using a diet that you can stick to permanently. There is some basis to support this approach. However, a very recent study[355] (May 2016) demonstrates that a diet alternating between low-carb/high-fat and a regular diet, is an effective strategy in controlling obesity, fatty liver, hyperinsulinemia and glucose intolerance, without even controlling caloric intake, making it an easily adoptable lifestyle modification. It shows that using any particular diet for long term enables the body to adapt and learn to utilize the macros more efficiently absorbing the maximum calories. By alternating one's diet between low-carb and moderate-carb, this study proves that the body is inefficient at absorbing the calories even while feeling satiated from the food we eat thus making it easier to lose weight. It's important to note that this study was done on mice; alternating from five days of low-carb to one day of regular diet did not demonstrate significant benefit; and alternating from five days of low-carb to two or five days of regular diet did demonstrate significant benefit. Further studies will be needed to determine the most beneficial alternation system in humans, and in all likelihood individual persons will react differently.

THE PHYSIOLOGY OF THE VERY LOW-CARBOHYDRATE DIET

The physiology of the very low-carbohydrate diet revolves around two primary guiding factors: blood sugar levels and liver glycogen levels.

Without carbohydrates in the diet, blood sugar levels drop. At first the body takes stored carbohydrates from the glycogen reserves in the liver to raise blood sugar levels to the healthy range that enables the body to function as required. Without carbohydrates in the diet to

---

355 Yongjie Ma, Mingming Gao, and Dexi Liu, "Alternating Diet as a Preventive and Therapeutic Intervention for High Fat Diet-induced Metabolic Disorder," *Scientific Reports*, May 18 2016, http://www.nature.com/articles/srep26325.

replenish the lowered glycogen reserves, the body begins to compensate for the lack of dietary carbohydrates via these two primary avenues:

1. Creating glucose by converting proteins and lipids into glucose (gluconeogenesis).
2. Relying upon lipids as a prime source of energy. Virtually all ingested lipids are used immediately upon absorption for fuel. Stored body fat is also released to be burned for fuel as necessary.

Some very low-carbohydrate diets exclude carbohydrates to such an extent that one does not get sufficient dietary fiber. The Dukan diet includes fiber supplements that have few calories. However, most experts recommend that fiber should be obtained through the consumption of foods, because they contain many micronutrients and bioactive compounds, which provide their own nutritional benefits. Dukan (in the induction phase) doesn't allow any carrots and red peppers—both are high in fiber and vitamin A, which are important vitamins in assisting with reducing fat cell numbers. And Atkins only allows twenty grams of carbohydrates total per day. Neither diet allows legumes, a cholesterol-free source of protein that is high in fiber and in important minerals, such as potassium, magnesium, iron, and zinc. In their strictest phases, these diets do not even allow green leafy vegetables (Atkins limits them to twenty grams), which are also high in fiber; vitamins A, B, C, and K; and minerals such as calcium.

On a very low-carbohydrate diet that includes fiber in foods such as those just listed, the carbohydrates ingested slow the fat-burning effects in the short term (compared to the Atkins and Dukan diets, which exclude such foods in their induction phase). However, the other nutrients these carbohydrates include will speed up fat loss in the long term.

Unless glycogen stores are full or nearly full, carbohydrates ingested will either be used immediately as fuel or stored as glycogen in the liver and muscle. *They won't be converted to fat for storage unless glycogen reserves are filled to capacity.*

GLYCOGEN RESERVE CAPACITY AND BODY-WEIGHT FLUCTUATION

The average person has nearly one pound of glycogen reserves, and three to four pounds of water is held with each pound of glycogen.[356] Muscle contains 1 to 2 percent glycogen, depending on conditioning (those who completely deplete and then completely refill their reserves have larger reserves than those who don't deplete their reserves). Since some people have considerably more muscle mass than others, their total glycogen reserves can be much higher than one pound; even more than two pounds.[357] Also, the estimate of three to four pounds of water stored within each pound of glycogen is disputed; some claim that the ratio is really 2.7:1, while others claim there isn't any consistent ratio at all.[358] An average person can gain or lose three to six pounds in glycogen/water fluctuation, while muscular athletes can gain or lose more than eleven pounds of glycogen/water reserves without changes in fat mass when reloading with carbohydrates after a low-carbohydrate diet or depleting filled reserves when beginning a low-carbohydrate diet.[359]

As an observant Jew, I honor the Sabbath with festive meals. For a twenty-four-hour period each week, I go off the restricted-carbohydrate diet. I enjoy fresh-baked bread, potatoes, cake, and even chocolate. If I entered the Sabbath while on the fat-loss diet, my glycogen reserves would be close to zero. Typically I am one to two pounds heavier Sunday morning than on the preceding Friday morning.

356   K. E. Olsson and B. Saltin, "Variation in Total Body Water with Muscle Glycogen Changes in Man," *Acta Physiologica Scandinavica* (September 1970), http://onlinelibrary.wiley.com/doi/10.1111/j.1748-1716.1970.tb04764.x/abstract;jsessionid=EFED180858B56C048802245B3A0F1E80.f02t04.

357   S. N. Kreitzman, A. Y. Coxon, and K. F. Szaz, "Glycogen Storage: Illusions of Easy Weight Loss, Excessive Weight Regain, and Distortions in Estimates of Body Composition," *American Journal of Clinical Nutrition* (July 1992) http://ajcn.nutrition.org/content/56/1/292S.long.

358   W. M. Sherman et al., "Muscle Glycogen Storage and Its Relationship with Water," *International Journal of Sports Medicine* (February 1982), http://www.ncbi.nlm.nih.gov/pubmed/7068293.

359   Kreitzman, Coxon, and Szaz, "Glycogen Storage."

However, that isn't fat gain but rather refilling the glycogen reserves plus the water that accompanies it. *The difference between two pounds of added glycogen stores and two pounds of fat is roughly the difference between one thousand and nine thousand calories, respectively.* Two pounds gained in glycogen reserves is about half a pound of glycogen and 1.5 pounds of water. Half a pound is almost 250 grams, and as each gram of glycogen stores four calories, hence the measurement of one thousand calories. Another way of calculating is that one gram of glycogen reserves equals one calorie, because glycogen reserves are one part glycogen and three parts water—every four grams of reserves has one gram of glycogen (and three grams of water) equal to four calories. A kilogram (one thousand grams) of glycogen reserves has one thousand calories. A kilogram of fat (2.2 pounds) is nine thousand calories (nine calories per gram). The added one thousand calories in the form of 2.2 pounds of filled glycogen reserves can be burned in two days of a five-hundred-calorie deficit. The same weight in fat, nine thousand calories, is obviously a much bigger project to burn off.

I mention my personal Sabbath customs because many people need an occasional break from the stress of restricted dieting, and it's important to understand what's happening inside us and how to make the best of the situation.

On the face of it, it appears that one day a week off the diet, requiring one to two days for recovery, might severely frustrate a fat-loss phase. But the situation of increased carbohydrates and insulin can be turned around to an *advantage!* Insulin becomes a major *liability* when glycogen reserves are full; the body is resistant to insulin, requiring larger doses to lower blood sugar, and since there is nowhere to store the sugar as glycogen, the insulin directs the liver to convert it to fat, which sends it through the blood for storage in fat cells—bad news.

However, when glycogen stores are low, insulin won't direct the liver to convert excess blood sugar into fat, and the body is more sensitive to insulin (lowering blood sugar quickly with just small amounts of insulin). Insulin becomes a major *asset*, one that potently speeds up nutrient absorption into all our cells. During the six carbohydrate-free days,

I have to minimize heavy muscle-building workouts, because without the carbohydrates and insulin, nutrition absorption is restricted, slowing down recovery. I save my heaviest lifting day for Friday and utilize my break from carbohydrate restriction for recovering from an intense workout. On the Sabbath, I make sure to ingest plenty of protein and food high in vitamins and minerals. With the added carbohydrates and the insulin, nutrient uptake is maximized.

Sundays and Mondays, I am extra careful about sticking with the Maimonides extended daily fast and use those mornings for long, intensive aerobic workouts before breakfast. This is crucial, because by Saturday night, my glycogen reserves are significantly fuller. Thus, to enable maximum fat loss during the coming week, I have to get those reserves back down near zero. *As you lower your glycogen reserves, the intensity of fat burning is increased.*[360] Maintaining low glycogen levels also protects us from fat accumulation when we temporarily slip off the diet. An ice cream cake eaten on full reserves is immediately converted to fat, leaving many people hungry soon after, but on empty reserves, it is stored as glycogen and more easily burned off.

By Monday or Tuesday morning, I usually get my weight down lower than it was the preceding Friday. But more importantly, by then I usually see progress in waist measurement. Since most of the glycogen reserves are in the muscles, even though the scales are telling me that I'm heavier on Sunday morning, there is barely any increase in waist measurement.

The goal on Sunday and Monday is not merely to get the glycogen levels back down for fat burning, but to utilize the increased stored energy for *longer and more intense workouts* that are not possible without glycogen. If that energy is applied to aerobics, doing intensive interval training (instead of merely burning off those carbohydrates with long slow aerobics) can *increase your aerobic capacity*, making future workouts more successful at burning off fat. If boosted glycogen energy is used for resistance training (during the maintenance or transition phase), you can benefit from muscle gain.

---

360   Katarina T. Borer, "Advanced Exercise Endocrinology," *Human Kinetics* (2013): 106.

RECORD PARAMETERS BEFORE
CHANGING YOUR DIET

Before making changes in your diet, it's important to measure and record your waistline, body weight, and certain blood levels. Since the vast majority of adults lack sufficient vitamin D, and since vitamin D is so important for health and fat-loss, you should pay close attention to your levels. If supplementation hasn't gotten your levels up sufficiently, you are not alone; for many people (especially overweight individuals) it takes mega doses of vitamin D supplements to reach sufficient levels.

- Waistline measurement: use a tape measure either at the height of your belly button or at the narrowest part (whichever you choose to measure, just be consistent about it to accurately measure changes). Women should also track their hip measurement at the widest point.
- Body weight: this should be measured in the morning for the most accurate record of body fat changes.
- Blood tests: use the chart below to track which levels to measure.

Diabetes risk parameters

Hemoglobin A1c	normal: 4–5.8%
Glucose	normal: 55–100 mg/dL
Fasting Insulin	too high: ≥25 mIU/L

Heart disease risk parameters

LDL	optimal ≤ 100
	near optimal 100–129
	borderline high 130–159
	high ≥ 160 mg/dL
HDL	low ≤ 40
	normal 40–60 mg/dL
Triglycerides	normal: ≤ 150 mg/dL
	borderline high 150-199 mg/dL

	high: 200-499 mg/dL
	very high: ≥500 mg/dL
Blood Pressure	normal: ≤120/80
	prehypertension: 120–129/80–89
	hypertension stage 1: 140–159/90–99
	hypertension stage 2: ≥160/100
	crisis: 180/110

	Key vitamins and minerals
Vitamin D	deficiency ≤ 10 ng/ml
	insufficiency 10–30
	sufficiency 30–100
	toxicity ≥ 100
Sodium	136–146 mmol/L
Potassium	3.5–5.1 mmol/L
Calcium	8.8–10.6 mg/dL

Once you have maintained dietary changes for a few months, you should periodically check (once every three to six months) the above, keeping track of your body's response to your lifestyle changes.

CONCLUDING SUMMARY

Permanent Diet and Exercise Policies
1. Finish dinner early
2. Do aerobic exercise before breakfast
3. Habituate to a late breakfast
4. Minimize nutrient-empty carbohydrates (sugar, refined grains, and potatoes)
5. Get sun exposure for vitamin D
6. Eat a high-protein and high-calcium diet that includes fish and high-protein, low-fat dairy
7. Eat a high-fiber diet
8. Perform resistance training in late afternoon
9. Make sure to get sufficient nutrients, specifically vitamin A, vitamin D, vitamin E, vitamin C, folate, calcium, magnesium, fiber, and potassium. Be wary of refined grains, added sugars, sodium, and saturated fat.
10. When eating meat and dairy products, opt for the grass-fed variety for the amazing benefits of CLA (conjugated linoleic acid).

Temporary High-Speed Fat-Loss Plan
1. Extreme reduction in carbs. Limit carbohydrates to high-fiber varieties (vegetables)
2. Minimal dietary fat
3. Unlimited protein
4. Continue with the permanent diet policies, with the exception of lighter exercise
5. Typically two to four weeks, with a gradual transition back to the permanent phase over an additional span of two to four weeks

Transitional Phase from Fat Loss to Permanent Policies
Gradually reintroduce carbohydrates (whole grains and potatoes), while gradually returning to more intensive exercise and heavier weight

lifting. Mildly restrict carbohydrates on most days, with one or two days per week nearly carbohydrate-free.

Take Advantage of Occasional Festive Meals

Work out heavily before the festive meal, and increase aerobic exercise the morning after.

Apply According to Your Individual Needs

Putting this information into practice is somewhat of a science and somewhat of an art—adapting to each individual's needs. The purpose of this book is not to replace the guidance of your dietitian or doctor but rather to give you the knowledge to make working with professional guidance more productive. Each person has his or her particular conditions and circumstances that can only be catered to on an individual basis by a qualified professional. Having this information available to review can spur on progress and help you maintain a lifelong commitment to a healthy lifestyle.

Wishing you success,
blessings, and health,

Yonason Herschlag

P. S. When I began writing this book I intended to include chapters on micronutrients and supplements for fat-loss and health, however, just getting through the macronutrients turned out to be a big enough project on its own. I have begun working on my next two books – one focused on micronutrients, and the next on the physiology of strength and body building, but I need your help. This book is a self-published effort; I focused on the content, not on marketing. Only if you my dear reader pass the word promoting this book to your friends and associates will enough sales be generated to enable me to stay focused on producing valuable content.

My congratulations to you for getting through this book; it's not light reading. You have proven to be seriously dedicated to the subject. By supporting me through promoting this book we can form a partnership in which I can continue to research and produce more books on this and related topics. I would greatly appreciate your review on Amazon; future potential readers depend on your feedback to decide on picking up the book. I also read the reviews and learn from them how to improve the next edition of this book and guide myself on additional books. You can also reach me at herschlag@012.net.il or yonasonherschlag@gmail. com ; I'm easier to communicate with than you might think.

Glossary

Adipose—fat tissue

ALA—alpha-linolenic acid; short-chain omega-3 fatty acid found in plants, such as flaxseed

Amino acid—class of organic compounds that contain at least one amino group, -NH2, and one carboxyl group, -COOH. The building blocks from which proteins are constructed

Atherosclerosis—a degenerative disease of the arteries characterized by patchy thickening of the inner lining of the arterial walls, caused by deposits of fatty material

ATP—adenosine triphosphate; intercellular fuel

Autophagy—the controlled destruction of damaged organelles within a cell

Apoptosis—a form of cell death in which a programmed sequence of events leads to the elimination of cells without releasing harmful substances into the surrounding area. Apoptosis plays a crucial role in developing and maintaining the health of the body by eliminating old cells, unnecessary cells, and unhealthy cells. The human body replaces perhaps one million cells per second.

BCAAs—branched chain amino acids; specifically, three amino acids: leucine, isoleucine, and valine. BCAAs are among the nine essential amino acids for humans, accounting for 35 percent of the essential amino acids in muscle tissue proteins. BCAAs are unique compared to all the seventeen other amino acids in that they can be oxidized/burned, in the muscle as fuel.

BMI—body mass index—to calculate BMI, divide your weight in kilograms (kg) by your height in meters (m), then divide the answer by your height again to get your BMI.

Catabolism—the process of breaking down chemical structures, usually for the purpose of harnessing life sustaining energy from them

Circadian rhythm—often referred to as the "body clock," the circadian rhythm is a twenty-four-hour cycle that tells our bodies when to sleep and regulates many other physiological processes. This internal body clock is affected by environmental cues, like sunlight and temperature.

Cholesterol—a soft waxy lipid found in animal cells and body fluids. Cholesterol is a special type of lipid that is called a steroid. Steroids are lipids that have a special chemical structure. This structure is made of four rings of carbon atoms. In fact, all steroid hormones are made from changing the basic chemical structure of cholesterol.

Cortisol—a hormone that triggers the liver to release stored fat and sugar into the blood and directs the liver to convert fats and proteins into sugar to further contribute to raising blood sugar levels. While affected slightly by stress and blood sugar levels, cortisol blood levels are dictated primarily by a circadian rhythm, which typically reaches a low point around midnight and its pinnacle at 8:30 a.m.

DHA—docosahexaenoic acid, a long-chain omega-3 fatty acid, plentiful in fish

Disaccharides—the sugars sucrose, lactose, and maltose; compounds with two carbohydrate molecules

Endothelium—the tissue that forms a single layer of cells lining various organs and cavities of the body, especially the blood vessels, heart, and lymphatic vessels

Enzyme—a chemical originating from living cells capable of causing chemical changes in organic substances by catalytic action, as in digestion

EPA—eicosapentaenoic acid; a long-chain omega-3 fatty acid, plentiful in fish

Fat cell—a cell that is specialized for the synthesis and storage of fat, otherwise known as an adipocyte

Fiber—the edible parts of plants or analogous carbohydrates that are resistant to digestion and absorption in the human small intestine, with complete or partial fermentation in the large intestine. It includes polysaccharides, oligosaccharides, lignin, and associated plant substances.

Ghrelin—a hormone that increases appetite via receptors in the hypothalamus and directs metabolism to store fat as opposed to burning it. Ghrelin also induces secretion of gastric acid and pancreatic enzymes, thereby increasing energy absorption.

Glycemic index—the *glycemic index*, or GI, ranks foods on a scale of 0–100 based on how quickly they raise blood sugar levels. Foods that raise blood sugar quickly have a higher number, whereas foods that take longer to raise blood sugar levels have a lower number. GI is categorized as either *low* (55 or less), *medium* (56–69), or *high* (70–100).

Glycemic load—the measurement of the glycemic index multiplied by the number of grams of carbohydrates ingested, divided by one hundred

Glucagon—a hormone formed in the pancreas that promotes the breakdown of glycogen to glucose in the liver

Gluconeogenesis—generating "new" glucose (primarily in the liver) from proteins and lipids

Glutamine—the most abundant amino acid in muscle and blood plasma. It is considered to be a nonessential amino acid because it is made by the body and is not absolutely required to be obtained through the diet. Although we do get glutamine in our diets, it is necessary for the body to produce more to meet the vast amounts required. Glutamine has many functions—one of which is being used for fuel in gluconeogenesis. Glutamine is also a primary source of fuel for the cells of the immune system

Glycogen—glucose is transformed by muscle and liver cells into a type of starch called glycogen for storage, hydrated with approximately three parts of water

Glycolysis—the breakdown of glucose by enzymes, releasing energy and pyruvic acid

HDL cholesterol—cholesterol can't dissolve in the blood. It must be transported through the bloodstream by carriers called lipoproteins (lipids encased in proteins). The two types of lipoproteins that carry cholesterol to and from cells are low-density lipoproteins, or LDLs, and high-density lipoproteins, or HDLs. HDL cholesterol is considered "good" cholesterol because, according to accepted theory, it helps remove LDL cholesterol from the arteries, carrying it to the liver, where it is broken down and passed out of the body.

Homeostatic Fat Mass Weight—the exact fat-mass weight that your body naturally stabilizes toward. Fat mass is maintained through compensating for changes in weight by adjusting the body's metabolic rate (rate of energy expenditure) and absorption of calories from digestion. When fat mass is suddenly reduced, the body slows energy expenditure and extracts more calories from digestion in attempt to return to the homeostatic fat mass weight

HGH—human growth hormone

HMG-CoA reductase—a liver enzyme that is responsible for producing cholesterol

Homeostasis—the tendency of a system to maintain internal stability, through the coordinated response of its parts, to situations or stimulus that would disturb its normal condition

Hormone—A chemical produced by living cells (usually a combination of amino acids forming a unique structure) that circulates in body fluids (primarily blood) and that triggers specific physiological reactions when contacting the receptors of other cells (often remote from its point of origin)

Hyperinsulinemia—an overabundance of insulin usually due to insulin resistance and high blood sugar

Hypothalamus—a small part of the brain located at its base that controls body temperature, hunger, thirst, fatigue, sleep, and more.

Insulin—a natural hormone made by the pancreas that controls the level of glucose in the blood. Insulin enables body cells to absorb and use glucose. Cells cannot utilize glucose without insulin.

Insulin resistance—one of the main functions of insulin is to transfer excess sugar from the blood into the liver and muscle cells; cells are said to be resistant to insulin when they resist the transfer of sugar

Insulin sensitivity—cells are said to be sensitive to insulin when they respond to insulin, accepting the transfer of sugar

In vitro—a biological process made to occur in a laboratory vessel as opposed in within a living organism

In vivo—a biological process made to occur within a living organism

Kabbalah—the mystical teachings of Judaism that delve into understanding the mystical spiritual forces that are the roots of the physical world

LDL cholesterol—LDL cholesterol is considered the "bad" cholesterol because it contributes to plaque, a thick, hard deposit that can clog arteries and make them less flexible. (See also *HDL cholesterol*)

Leptin—a hormone that suppresses appetite via the receptors in the hypothalamus and increases energy expenditure by burning more fat, leading to a reduction in the body weight and adiposity

Lipogenesis—fat creation. The process by which the liver converts excess sugar into fat for storage

Lipolysis—fat breakdown. The biochemical pathway responsible for the catabolism of triacylglycerol (TAG) stored in cellular lipid droplets enabling its use for energy

Macronutrients—nutrients (required in large amounts compared to micronutrients) that provide calories or energy: carbohydrates, proteins, and fats

Metabolism—includes the metabolic processes of anabolism and catabolism. Anabolism is the process of building biochemical structures for a broad array of functions that the body needs to maintain life

Metabolic syndrome—a combination of obesity and high cholesterol, high blood pressure, and high blood sugar that increases the risk of heart disease, cancer, and diabetes, some of the leading causes of death. The prevalence of this syndrome is estimated to be between 20 to 25 percent of adult Americans

Micronutrients—dietary components not produced in the body and which must be derived from the diet, often referred to as vitamins and minerals, which—although only required by the body in small amounts relative to macronutrients—are vital to development, disease prevention, and overall health

Mitochondria—structures inside cells that utilize glucose, fatty acids, and some amino acids combined with oxygen to generate ATP, the body's cellular fuel

Monosaccharides—simple sugars including glucose, fructose, and galactose; carbohydrate compounds having just one carbohydrate molecule

Paleo—prehistoric

Paleo diet—mimics the diet that evolutionists theorize prehistoric humans ate

Polysaccharides—a carbohydrate (e.g., starch, cellulose, or glycogen) whose molecules consist of a number of sugar molecules bonded together

Prediabetes—a condition of high glucose levels that are not as so high to be classified as diabetes

Saccharides—carbohydrates consisting of *monosaccharides, disaccharides,* and *polysaccharides.* Carbohydrate compounds having just one carbohydrate molecule are called *monosaccharides.* Compounds with two carbohydrate molecules are called *disaccharides,* and compounds containing at least three (sometimes as many as sixty thousand) carbohydrate molecules are named *polysaccharides.*

Talmud—the ancient oral traditions concerning Jewish law and study. After the destruction of the second temple in Jerusalem, the sages decided to compile the oral traditions into a written form so they shouldn't be forgotten. The first stage of this was the compilation of the Mishna around eighteen hundred years ago, which is a summary of the oral teachings. About two hundred years later, the Gemara (also referred to as the Talmud), which expounds on the Mishna, was compiled by the leading sages so that the teachings would be preserved. The Talmud is comprised of sixty-three tractates and is approximately sixty-two hundred pages long. It is written in a mixture of Hebrew and Aramaic.

Talmudist—a student of the Talmud

Thermogenesis—the burning of calories via the genesis, or creation, of body heat

Treifa—a Hebrew word meaning a torn animal

Triglyceride—a type of fat used to store excess energy from the diet. High levels of triglycerides in the blood are associated with atherosclerosis. Elevated triglycerides can be caused by obesity, physical inactivity, cigarette smoking, excess alcohol consumption, and a diet high in carbohydrates

Bibliography

Books; English

American Heart Association. *The No-Fad Diet.* 2011.

Atkins. *Dr. Atkins' New Diet Revolution.* New York: HarperCollins Publishers, 2002.

Borer. *Advanced Exercise Endocrinology.* Human Kinetics. 2013.

Cordain. *The Paleo Diet: Lose Weight and Get Healthy by Eating the Foods You Were Designed to Eat.* New York, NY: Houghton Mifflin Harcourt, 2011.

Darwin. *The Origin of Species by Means of Natural Selection, or the Preservation of Favoured Races in the Struggle for Life.* 6th ed. London: John Murray, 1876.

Dukan. *The Dukan Diet.* Hodder and Stoughton, 2010.

Fuhrman. *Eat to Live: The Amazing Nutrient-Rich Program for Fast and Sustained Weight Loss.* New York: Little Brown, 2011.

Gould. *The Panda's Thumb.*

Gropper, Smith, and Groff. *Advanced Nutrition and Human Metabolism.* 5th ed. Cengage Learning, 2008.

Guyton and Hall. *Textbook of Medical Physiology.* Saunders, 2011.

Holick. *The Vitamin D Solution.* Hudson Street Press, 2010.

Institute of Medicine. *Dietary Reference Intakes.* National Academies Press, 2005.

Macdonald. *Body Confidence.* HarperCollins, 2011.

Rosner. "The Life of Moses Maimonides: Prominent Medieval Physician." *Einstein Quartet Journal of Biology and Medicine* (2002).

Sears. *Enter the Zone.* HarperCollins, 1995.

Zaklikowski. *Maimonides: His Life and Works.*

Books; Hebrew

Avli. *Magen Avraham.* Aruch Chaim, Chapter 157.

Ben-Asher. *Tur.* Aruch Chaim, Chapter 155.

Epstein. *Meor VaShemesh.* 1822.

Kairo. *Shulchan Aruch.* Aruch Chaim, Chapter 157.

Kegan. *Mishna Brura.* Aruch Chaim Chapter 157.

Maimonides. *Mishneh Torah, Kedusha* (Holiness), hilchot machlot is-surot (laws of forbidden foods), chapter 4.

Maimonides. *Mishneh Torah, HaMada* (Knowledge), hilchat Dayot, chapter 4.

Talmud Tractate, Pesachim.

Talmud Tractate, Rosh HaShona.

Talmud Tractate, Shabbas.

Talmud Tractate, Succah.

Yitzchaki. *Rashi*. Talmud Tractate Succah.

Studies; Diet

Abete, Parra, de Morentin, and Martinez. "Effects of Two Energy-Restricted Diets Differing in the Carbohydrate/Protein Ratio on Weight Loss and Oxidative Changes of Obese Men." *International Journal of Food Sciences and Nutrition* (2009). http://www.ncbi.nlm. nih.gov/pubmed/18654910.

Astrup. "The Satiating Power of Protein: A Key to Obesity Prevention?" *American Journal of Clinical Nutrition* (2005). http://ajcn.nutrition. org/content/82/1/1.full.

Bailes, Strow, Werthammer, McGinnis, and Elitsur. "Effect of Low-Carbohydrate, Unlimited Calorie Diet on the Treatment of Childhood Obesity: A Prospective Controlled Study." *Metabolic Syndrome and Related Disorders* (2003). http://www.ncbi.nlm.nih. gov/pubmed/18370665.

Bilsborough and Mann. "A Review of Issues of Dietary Protein Intake in Humans." *International Journal of Sport Nutrition and Exercise Metabolism* (2006). http://www.ncbi.nlm.nih.gov/ pubmed/16779921.

Brehm, Seeley, Daniels, and D'Alessio. "A Randomized Trial Comparing a Very Low Carbohydrate Diet and a Calorie-Restricted Low Fat Diet on Body Weight and Cardiovascular Risk Factors in Healthy Women." *Journal of Clinical Endocrinology and*

Metabolism (2003). http://press.endocrine.org/doi/full/10.1210/jc.2002-021480.

Bueno, de Melo, de Oliveira, and da Rocha. "Very-Low-Carbohydrate Ketogenic Diet v. Low-Fat Diet for Long-Term Weight Loss: A Meta-Analysis of Randomised Controlled Trials." *British Journal of Nutrition* (2013). http://www.ncbi.nlm.nih.gov/pubmed/23651522.

Cahill, Chiuve, Mekary, Jensen, Flint, Hu, and Rimm. "Prospective Study of Breakfast Eating and Incident Coronary Heart Disease in a Cohort of Male US Health Professionals." *Circulation* 128 (2013): 337–43. http://circ.ahajournals.org/content/128/4/337.full.pdf.

Cao and Nielsen. "Acid Diet (High-Meat Protein) Effects on Calcium Metabolism and Bone Health." *Current Opinion in Clinical Nutrition and Metabolic Care* (2010). http://www.ncbi.nlm.nih.gov/pubmed/20717017.

Carlson and Hoelzel. "Apparent Prolongation of the Life Span of Rats by Intermittent Fasting." *Journal of Nutrition* (1946), http://www.ncbi.nlm.nih.gov/pubmed/21021020..

Daly, Paisey, Millward, Eccles, Williams, Hammersley, MacLeod, and Gale. "Short-Term Effects of Severe Dietary Carbohydrate-Restriction Advice in Type 2 Diabetes." *Diabetic Medicine* (2006). http://www.ncbi.nlm.nih.gov/pubmed/16409560.

Christopher D. Gardner et al.. "Comparison of the Atkins, Zone, Ornish, and Learn Diets for Change in Weight and Related Risk Factors among Overweight Premenopausal Women: The A to Z Weight Loss Study." *Journal of the American Medical Association* (2007). http://jama.jamanetwork.com/article.aspx?articleid=205916.

Dyson, Beatty, and Matthew. "A Low-Carbohydrate Diet Is More Effective in Reducing Body Weight than Healthy Eating in Both Diabetic and Non-Diabetic Subjects." *Diabetic Medicine* (2007). http://www.ncbi.nlm.nih.gov/pubmed/17971178.

Foster, Wyatt, Hill, McGuckin, Brill, Mohammed, Szapary, Rader, Edman, and Klein. "A Randomized Trial of a Low-Carbohydrate Diet for Obesity." *New England Journal of Medicine* (2003). http://www.nejm.org/doi/full/10.1056/NEJMoa022207#t=articleMethods.

Gannon and Nuttall. "Effect of a High-Protein, Low-Carbohydrate Diet on Blood Glucose Control in People with Type 2 Diabetes." *Diabetes* (2004).

Gardner, Kiazand, Alhassan, Kim, Stafford, Balise, Kraemer, and King. "Comparison of the Atkins, Zone, Ornish, and Learn Diets for Change in Weight and Related Risk Factors among Overweight Premenopausal Women: The A to Z Weight Loss Study." *Journal of the American Medical Association* (2007). http://jama.jamanetwork.com/article.aspx?articleid=205916.

Halberg, Henriksen, Söderhamn, Stallknecht, Ploug, Schjerling, and Dela. "Effect of Intermittent Fasting and Refeeding on Insulin Action in Healthy Men." *Journal of Applied Physiology* 99, no. 6 (December 2005): 2128–36. http://jap.physiology.org/content/99/6/2128

Halton and Hu. "The Effects of High Protein Diets on Thermogenesis, Satiety and Weight Loss: A Critical Review." *Journal of the American College of Nutrition* (2004). http://www.colorado.edu/intphys/Class/IPHY3700_Greene/pdfs/discussionEssay/thermogenesisSatiety/HaltonProtein2004.pdf.

Harvie, Pegington, Mattson, Frystyk, Dillon, Evans, Cuzick, et al. "The Effects of Intermittent or Continuous Energy Restriction on Weight Loss and Metabolic Disease Risk Markers: A Randomised Trial in Young Overweight Women." *International Journal of Obesity* (May 2011). http://www.ncbi.nlm.nih.gov/pmc/articles/PMC3017674/.

Hatori, Megumi et al. "Time-Restricted Feeding without Reducing Caloric Intake Prevents Metabolic Diseases in Mice Fed a High-Fat Diet." *Cell Metabolism* 15, no. 6 (June 6, 2012). 848–60. http://www.cell.com/cell-metabolism/abstract/S1550-4131(12)00189-1.

Heilbronn, Smith, Martin, Anton, and Ravussin. "Alternate-Day Fasting in Nonobese Subjects: Effects on Body Weight, Body Composition, and Energy Metabolism." *American Journal of Clinical Nutrition* (2005). http://ajcn.nutrition.org/content/81/1/69.full.pdf+html.

Hession, Rolland, Kulkarni, Wise, and Broom. "Systematic Review of Randomized Controlled Trials of Low-Carbohydrate vs. Low-Fat/Low-Calorie Diets in the Management of Obesity and Its Comorbidities." *Obesity Reviews* (2009). http://onlinelibrary.wiley.com/doi/10.1111/j.1467-789X.2008.00518.x/pdf.

Holt, Miller, Petocz, and Farmakalidis. "A Satiety Index of Common Foods." *European Journal of Clinical Nutrition* (1995). http://www.ncbi.nlm.nih.gov/pubmed/7498104.

Hu, Manson, Stampfer, Colditz, Liu, Solomon, and Willett. "Diet, Lifestyle, and the Risk of Type 2 Diabetes Mellitus in Women." *New England Journal of Medicine* (2001). http://www.nejm.org/doi/full/10.1056/NEJMoa010492.

Labayen, Díez, González, Parra, and Martínez. "Effects of Protein vs. Carbohydrate-Rich Diets on Fuel Utilisation in Obese Women during Weight Loss." *Forum of Nutrition* (2003). http://www.ncbi. nlm.nih.gov/pubmed/15806847.

Layman, Evans, Erickson, Seyler, Weber, Bagshaw, Griel, Psota, and Etherton. "A Moderate-Protein Diet Produces Sustained Weight Loss and Long-Term Changes in Body Composition and Blood Lipids in Obese Adults." *Journal of Nutrition* (2009). http:// jn.nutrition.org/content/139/3/514.long.

Leidy, Tang, Armstrong, Martin, and Campbell. "The Effects of Consuming Frequent, Higher Protein Meals on Appetite and Satiety during Weight Loss in Overweight/Obese Men." *Obesity* (2011). http://www.ncbi.nlm.nih.gov/pubmed/20847729

Lepe, Bacardí Gascón, and Jiménez Cruz. "Long-Term Efficacy of High-Protein Diets: A Systematic Review." *Nutrición Hospitalaria* (2011). http://www.ncbi.nlm.nih.gov/pubmed/22411369.

Little and Feinle-Bisset. "Effects of Dietary Fat on Appetite and Energy Intake in Health and Obesity—Oral and Gastrointestinal Sensory Contributions." *Physiology and Behavior* (2011). http://www.ncbi. nlm.nih.gov/pubmed/21596051.

McAuley, Hopkins, Smith, McLay, Williams, Taylor, and Mann. "Comparison of High-Fat and High-Protein Diets with a High-Carbohydrate Diet in Insulin-Resistant Obese Women." *Diabetologia* (2005). http://www.ncbi.nlm.nih.gov/ pubmed/15616799.

Mekary, Giovannucci, Willett, van Dam, and Hu. "Eating Patterns and Type 2 Diabetes Risk in Men: Breakfast Omission, Eating Frequency, and Snacking." *American Journal of Clinical Nutrition* (2012). http://ajcn.nutrition.org/content/95/5/1182.full.

Nickols-Richardson, Coleman, Volpe, and Hosig. "Perceived Hunger Is Lower and Weight Loss Is Greater in Overweight Premenopausal Women Consuming a Low-Carbohydrate/High-Protein vs. High-Carbohydrate/Low-Fat Diet." *Journal of the American Dietetic Association* (2005). http://www.nel.gov/worksheet. cfm?worksheet_id=250712.

Pereira, Swain, Goldfine, Rifai, and Ludwig. "Effects of a Low-Glycemic Load Diet on Resting Energy Expenditure and Heart Disease Risk Factors during Weight Loss." *Journal of the American Medical Association* (2004). http://www.ncbi.nlm.nih.gov/ pubmed/15562127.

Samaha, Iqbal, Seshadri, Chicano, Daily, McGrory, Williams, Williams, Gracely, and Stern. "A Low-Carbohydrate as Compared with a Low-Fat Diet in Severe Obesity." *New England Journal of Medicine* (2003). http://www.nejm.org/doi/full/10.1056/NEJMoa022637.

Santesso, Akl, Bianchi, Mente, Mustafa, Heels-Ansdell, and Schünemann. "Effects of Higher- versus Lower-Protein Diets on Health Outcomes: A Systematic Review and Meta-Analysis." *European Journal of Clinical Nutrition* (2012). http://www.nature. com/ejcn/journal/v66/n7/full/ejcn201237a.html.

Saslow, Kim, Daubenmier, Moskowitz, Phinney, Goldman, et al. "A Randomized Pilot Trial of a Moderate Carbohydrate Diet Compared with a Very Low Carbohydrate Diet in Overweight or Obese Individuals with Type 2 Diabetes Mellitus or Prediabetes." *PLoS One* 9 (2014).

Schwingshackl and Hoffmann. "Long-Term Effects of Low-Fat Diets Either Low or High in Protein on Cardiovascular and Metabolic

Risk Factors: A Systematic Review and Meta-Analysis." *Nutrition Journal* (2013). http://www.biomedcentral.com/content/pdf/1475-2891-12-48.pdf.

Shai, et al., "Weight Loss with a Low-Carbohydrate, Mediterranean, or Low-Fat Diet." *New England Journal of Medicine* (2008). http://www.nejm.org/doi/full/10.1056/NEJMoa0708681.

Skov, Toubro, Rùnn, Holm, and Astrup. "Randomized Trial on Protein vs. Carbohydrate in Ad Libitum Fat Reduced Diet for the Treatment of Obesity." *International Journal of Obesity* (1999). http://www.ncbi.nlm.nih.gov/pubmed/10375057.

Sondike, Copperman, and Jacobson. "Effects of A Low-Carbohydrate Diet on Weight Loss and Cardiovascular Risk Factor in Overweight Adolescents." *Journal of Pediatrics* (2003). http://www.ncbi.nlm.nih.gov/pubmed/12640371.

Tsigris. "Review of Long-Term Weight Loss Results after Laparoscopic Sleeve Gastrectomy." *Journal of Surgery for Obesity and Related Diseases* 10, no. 1 (January/February 2014): 177–183. http://www.soard.org/article/S1550-7289(13)00381-X/fulltext.

Van der Heijden, Hu, Rimm, and van Dam. "A Prospective Study of Breakfast Consumption and Weight Gain among US Men." *Obesity* (2007). http://onlinelibrary.wiley.com/doi/10.1038/oby.2007.292/full.

Varady, Bhutani, Church, and Klempel. "Short-Term Modified Alternate-Day Fasting: A Novel Dietary Strategy for Weight Loss and Cardioprotection in Obese Adults." *American Journal of Clinical Nutrition* (2009). http://ajcn.nutrition.org/content/90/5/1138.

Volek, Phinney, Forsythe, Quann, Wood, Puglisi, Kraemer, et al. "Carbohydrate Restriction Has a More Favorable Impact on the Metabolic Syndrome than a Low Fat Diet." *Lipids* (2009). http://link.springer.com/article/10.1007/s11745-008-3274-2/fulltext.html.

Volek, Sharman, Gómez, Judelson, Rubin, Watson, Sokmen, Silvestre, French, and Kraemer. "Comparison of Energy-Restricted Very-Low-Carbohydrate and Low-Fat Diets on Weight Loss and Body Composition in Overweight Men and Women." *Nutrition and Metabolism* (2004). http://www.ncbi.nlm.nih.gov/pmc/articles/PMC538279/#B9.

Wady Aude, Agatston, Lopez-Jimenez, Lieberman, Almon, Hansen, Rojas, Lamas, and Hennekens. "The National Cholesterol Education Program Diet vs. a Diet Lower in Carbohydrates and Higher in Protein and Monounsaturated Fat." *Archives of Internal Medicine* (2004). http://archinte.jamanetwork.com/article.aspx?articleid=217514.

Walker Lasker, Evans, and Layman. "Moderate Carbohydrate, Moderate Protein Weight Loss Diet Reduces Cardiovascular Disease Risk Compared to High Carbohydrate, Low Protein Diet in Obese Adults: A Randomized Clinical Trial." *Nutrition and Metabolism* (2008). http://www.nutritionandmetabolism.com/content/5/1/30.

Westman, Yancy Jr., Mavropoulos, Marquart, and McDuffie. "The Effect of a Low-Carbohydrate, Ketogenic Diet versus a Low-Glycemic Index Diet on Glycemic Control in Type 2 Diabetes Mellitus." *Nutrition and Metabolism* (2008). http://www.ncbi.nlm.nih.gov/pmc/articles/PMC2633336/.

Yancy Jr., Foy, Chalecki, Vernon, and Westman. "A Low-Carbohydrate, Ketogenic Diet to Treat Type 2 Diabetes." *Nutrition and Metabolism* (2005). http://www.nutritionandmetabolism.com/content/2/1/34.

Yancy Jr., Olsen, Guyton, Bakst, E. C. Westman. "A Low-Carbohydrate, Ketogenic Diet versus a Low-Fat Diet to Treat Obesity and Hyperlipidemia." *Annals of Internal Medicine* (2004). http://www.ncbi.nlm.nih.gov/pubmed/15148063.

Yongjie, Mingming, and Dexi. "Alternating Diet as a Preventive and Therapeutic Intervention for High Fat Diet-induced Metabolic Disorder," *Scientific Reports*, May 18, 2016. http://www.nature.com/articles/srep26325.

Young, Scanlan, Im, and Lutwak. "Effect of Body Composition and Other Parameters in Obese Young Men of Carbohydrate Level of Reduction Diet." *American Journal of Clinical Nutrition* (1971). http://ajcn.nutrition.org/content/24/3/290.full.pdf+html.

Studies; Diet; Calcium, Vitamins D and A

Alvarez and Ashraf. "Role of Vitamin D in Insulin Secretion and Insulin Sensitivity for Glucose Homeostasis." *International Journal of Endocrinology* (2010). http://www.ncbi.nlm.nih.gov/pmc/articles/PMC2778451/.

Bolland, Avenell, Baron, Grey, MacLennan, Gamble, and Reid. "Effect of Calcium Supplements on Risk of Myocardial Infarction and Cardiovascular Events: Meta-Analysis." *BMJ* (December 2010). http://www.bmj.com/content/341/bmj.c3691

Jeyakumar, Vajreswari, Sesikeran, and Giridharan. "Vitamin A Supplementation Induces Adipose Tissue Loss through Apoptosis in Lean but Not in Obese Rats of the WNIN/OB Strain." *Journal of Molecular Endocrinology* (October 1, 2005). http://jme.endocrinology-journals.org/content/35/2/391.full.

Paik, Curhan, Sun, Rexrode, Manson, Rimm, and Taylor. "Calcium Supplement Intake and Risk of Cardiovascular Disease in Women." *Osteoporosis International* (August 2014). http://www.ncbi.nlm.nih.gov/pmc/articles/PMC4102630/.

Schrager. "Dietary Calcium Intake and Obesity." *Journal of the American Board of Family Medicine* (May 2005). http://www.jabfm.org/content/18/3/205.full.

Sergeev and Song. "High Vitamin D and Calcium Intakes Reduce Diet-Induced Obesity in Mice by Increasing Adipose Tissue Apoptosis." *Molecular Nutrition and Food Research* (June 2014). http://www.ncbi.nlm.nih.gov/pubmed/24449427.

Shapses, Heshka, and Heymsfield. "Effect of Calcium Supplementation on Weight and Fat Loss in Women." *Journal of Clinical Endocrinology and Metabolism*. (February 2004). http://www.ncbi.nlm.nih.gov/pubmed/14764774

Soheilykhah. "The Role of Adipocyte Mediators, Inflammatory Markers and Vitamin D in Gestational Diabetes." *Intech* (November 2011). http://cdn.intechopen.com/pdfs-wm/23178.pdf.

Sun and Zemel. "Role of Uncoupling Protein 2 (UCP 2) Expression and 1Alpha, 25-Dihydroxyvitamin D3 in Modulating Adipocyte Apoptosis." *FASEB Journal* (September 2004). http://www.ncbi.nlm.nih.gov/pubmed/15231722.

Talaei, Mohamadi, and Adgi. "The Effect of Vitamin D on Insulin Resistance in Patients with Type 2 Diabetes." *Diabetology and Metabolic Syndrome* (2013). http://www.dmsjournal.com/content/5/1/8.

Vigna et al. "Vitamin D Supplementation Promotes Weight Loss and Waist Circumference Reduction in Overweight/Obese Adults with Hypovitaminosis D," Presented at: European Congress on Obesity. (May 2015); Prague. http://www.clinicaladvisor.com/web-exclusives/vitamin-d-weight-loss-obese-overweight-deficiency/article/413772/

Zemel. "Regulation of Adiposity and Obesity Risk by Dietary Calcium: Mechanisms and Implications." *Journal of the American College of Nutrition* (April 2002). http://www.ncbi.nlm.nih.gov/pubmed/11999543.

Studies; Diet; CLA

Białek, Tokarz. "Conjugated Linoleic Acid as a Potential Protective Factor in Prevention of Breast Cancer." *Postępy higieny i medycyny doświadczalnej* (January 2013). http://www.ncbi.nlm.nih.gov/pubmed/23475478

Blankson, Stakkestad, Fagertun, Thom, Wadstein, and Gudmundsen. "Conjugated Linoleic Acid Reduces Body Fat Mass in Overweight and Obese Humans." *Journal of Nutrition* (June 2000). http://jn.nutrition.org/content/130/12/2943.short.

Castro-Webb, Ruiz-Narváez, and Campos. "Cross-Sectional Study of Conjugated Linoleic Acid in Adipose Tissue and Risk of Diabetes," *American Journal of Clinical Nutrition* (July 1996). http://www.ncbi.nlm.nih.gov/pubmed/22648724

Chen, Lin, Huang, Hsu, Houng, Huang. "Effect of conjugated Linoleic Acid Supplementation on Weight Loss and Body Fat Composition in a Chinese Population." *Nutrition* (May 2012). http://www.ncbi.nlm.nih.gov/pubmed/22261578.

Steck, Chalecki, P. Miller, Conway, Austin, Hardin, Albright, and Thuillier. "Conjugated Linoleic Acid Supplementation for Twelve Weeks Increases Lean Body Mass in Obese Humans." *Journal of Nutrition* (May 2007). http://www.ncbi.nlm.nih.gov/pubmed/17449580.

Watras, Buchholz, Close, Zhang, and Schoeller. "The Role of Conjugated Linoleic Acid in Reducing Body Fat and Preventing Holiday Weight Gain," *International Journal of Obesity* (March 2007). http://www.ncbi.nlm.nih.gov/pubmed/16924272.

Studies; Diet; Fiber

Abrams, Griffin, Hawthorne, Liang, Gunn, Darlington, and Ellis. "A Combination of Prebiotic Short- and Long-Chain Inulin-Type Fructans Enhances Calcium Absorption and Bone Mineralization in Young Adolescents." *American Journal of Clinical Nutrition* (2005). http://www.ncbi.nlm.nih.gov/pubmed/16087995.

Coudray, Demigné, and Rayssiguier. "Effects of Dietary Fibers on Magnesium Absorption in Animals and Humans." *Journal of Nutrition* (2003). http://www.ncbi.nlm.nih.gov/pubmed/12514257.

Edwards, Johnson, and Read. "Do Viscous Polysaccharides Slow Absorption by Inhibiting Diffusion or Convection?" *European Journal of Clinical Nutrition* (April 1988). http://www.ncbi.nlm.nih.gov/pubmed/2840277.

Greger. "Nondigestible Carbohydrates and Mineral Bioavailability." *Journal of Nutrition* (1999). http://jn.nutrition.org/content/129/7/1434S.full.

Johnston, Thomas, Bell, Frost, and Robertson. "Resistant Starch Improves Insulin Sensitivity in Metabolic Syndrome." *Diabetic Medicine* (2010). http://www.ncbi.nlm.nih.gov/pubmed/20536509.

Ladislav and Hannelore. "Mechanisms Underlying the Effects of Inulin-Type Fructans on Calcium Absorption in the Large Intestine of Rats." *Bone* 37, no. 5 (November 2005): 728–35. http://www.the-bonejournal.com/article/S8756-3282(05)00249-8/abstract.

Robertson, Currie, Morgan, Jewell, and Frayn. "Prior Short-Term Consumption of Resistant Starch Enhances Postprandial Insulin Sensitivity in Healthy Subjects." *Diabetologia* 46, no. 5 (May 2003): 659–65. http://link.springer.com/article/10.1007%2Fs00125-003-1081-0.

Scholz-Ahrens and Schrezenmeir. "Inulin and Oligofructose and Mineral Metabolism: The Evidence from Animal Trials." *Journal of Nutrition* (2007). http://www.ncbi.nlm.nih.gov/pubmed/17951495.

Tako, Glahn, Welch, Lei, Yasuda, and Miller. "Dietary Inulin Affects the Expression of Intestinal Enterocyte Iron Transporters, Receptors and Storage Protein and Alters the Microbiota in the Pig Intestine." *British Journal of Nutrition* (2008). http://www.ncbi.nlm.nih.gov/pubmed/17868492.

Zhang, Wang, Zhang, and Yang. "Effects of Resistant Starch on Insulin Resistance of Type 2 Diabetes Mellitus Patients." *Zhonghua Yu Fang Yi Xue Za Zhi* (2007). http://www.ncbi.nlm.nih.gov/pubmed/17605234.

Studies; Diet; Lipids

Ahmadvand, Mabuchi, Nohara, Kobayahi, and Kawashiri. "Effects of Coenzyme Q(10) on LDL Oxidation in Vitro." *Acta medica Iranica* (2013). http://www.ncbi.nlm.nih.gov/pubmed/23456579.

Al-Ghamdi, Jiman-Fatani, and El-Banna. "Role of Chlamydia Pneumoniae, Helicobacter Pylori and Cytomegalovirus in Coronary Artery Disease." *Pakistan Journal of Pharmaceutical Sciences* (April 24, 2011). http://www.ncbi.nlm.nih.gov/pubmed/21454155.

Assunção, Ferreira, dos Santos, Cabral Jr, and Florêncio. "Effects of Dietary Coconut Oil on the Biochemical and Anthropometric Profiles of Women Presenting Abdominal Obesity." *Lipids* (July 2009). http://www.ncbi.nlm.nih.gov/pubmed/19437058.

Bassett, Edel, Patenaude, McCullough, Blackwood, Chouinard, Paquin, Lamarche, and Pierce. "Dietary Vaccenic Acid Has Antiatherogenic Effects in LDLr-/- Mice." *Journal of Nutrition* (2010). http://jn.nutrition.org/content/140/1/18.

Bazian. "Saturated Fats and Heart Disease Link 'Unproven,'" *Behind the Headlines*, Health News from NHS Choices (March 18, 2014). http://www.nhs.uk/news/2014/03march/pages/saturated-fats-and-heart-disease-link-unproven.aspx

Chowdhury, Warnakula, Kunutsor, Crowe, Ward, Johnson, Franco, et al. "Association of Dietary, Circulating, and Supplement Fatty Acids with Coronary Risk: A Systematic Review and Meta-Analysis." *Annals of Internal Medicine* 160, no. 6 (March 18, 2014). http://annals.org/article.aspx?articleid=1846638.

Dulloo, Fathi, Mensi, and Girardier. "Twenty-Four-Hour Energy Expenditure and Urinary Catecholamines of Humans Consuming Low-to-Moderate Amounts of Medium-Chain Triglycerides: A Dose-Response Study in a Human Respiratory Chamber." *European Journal of Clinical Nutrition* (March 1996). http://www.ncbi.nlm. nih.gov/pubmed/8654328.

Duntas. "Thyroid Disease and Lipids." *Thyroid* (April 12, 2002). http:// www.ncbi.nlm.nih.gov/pubmed/12034052.

Kabara, Swieczkowski, Conley, and Truant. "Fatty Acids and Derivatives as Antimicrobial Agents." *Antimicrobial Agents and Chemotherapy* (July 1972). http://www.ncbi.nlm.nih.gov/pmc/articles/PMC444260/.

Kim, Jeon, Park, Choi, Kang, and Min. "Helicobacter Pylori Infection is Associated with Elevated Low Density Lipoprotein Cholesterol Levels in Elderly Koreans." *Journal of Korean Medical Science* (May 2011). http://www.ncbi.nlm.nih.gov/pmc/articles/PMC3082118/.

Legrand and Rioux. "The Complex and Important Cellular and Metabolic Functions of Saturated Fatty Acids." *Lipids* (July 13, 2010). http://www.ncbi.nlm.nih.gov/pmc/articles/PMC2974191/.

Liau, Lee, Chen, and Rasool. "An Open-Label Pilot Study to Assess the Efficacy and Safety of Virgin Coconut Oil in Reducing Visceral Adiposity." *ISRN Pharmacology* (2011). http://www.ncbi.nlm.nih. gov/pmc/articles/PMC3226242/.

Liberopoulos and Elisaf. "Dyslipidemia in Patients with Thyroid Disorders." *Hormones* (2002). http://www.hormones.gr/31/article/ article.html.

Mensink and Katan. "Effect of Dietary Trans Fatty Acids on High-Density and Low-Density Lipoprotein Cholesterol Levels in Healthy Subjects." *New England Journal of Medicine* (August 1990). http://www.ncbi.nlm.nih.gov/pubmed/2374566.

Mensink and Katan. "Effect of Dietary Fatty Acids on Serum Lipids and Lipoproteins: A Meta-Analysis of 27 Trials." *Arteriosclerosis and Thrombosis: A Journal of Vascular Biology* (August 1992). http://atvb.aha-journals.org/content/12/8/911.full.pdf?origin=publication_detail.

Nicolosi. "Dietary Fat Saturation Effects on Low-Density-Lipoprotein Concentrations and Metabolism in Various Animal Models." *American Journal of Clinical Nutrition* 65, no. 5 (1997). http://ajcn.nutrition.org/content/65/5/1617S.abstract.

Ogbolu, Oni, Daini, and Oloko. "In Vitro Antimicrobial Properties of Coconut Oil on Candida Species in Ibadan, Nigeria." *Journal of Medicinal Food* (June 2007). http://www.ncbi.nlm.nih.gov/pubmed/17651080.

Packard, McKinney, Carr, and Shepherd. "Cholesterol Feeding Increases Low Density Lipoprotein Synthesis." *Journal of Clinical Investigation* (July 1983). http://www.ncbi.nlm.nih.gov/pmc/articles/PMC1129159/.

Rioux and Legrand. "Saturated Fatty Acids: Simple Molecular Structures with Complex Cellular Functions." *Current Opinion in Clinical Nutrition and Metabolic Care* (2007).

Rtubbs and Harbron. "Covert Manipulation of the Ratio of Medium- to Long-Chain Triglycerides in Isoenergetically Dense Diets: Effect on Food Intake in Ad Libitum Feeding Men," *International Journal of Obesity and Related Metabolic Disorders* (May 1996). http://www.ncbi.nlm.nih.gov/pubmed/8696422.

Saada, Mekky, Eldawy, and Abdelaal. "Biological Effect of Sucralose in Diabetic Rats." *Food and Nutrition Sciences* 4, no. 7A (July 2013). http://www.scirp.org/journal/PaperInformation.aspx?PaperID=34006.

Scalfi, Coltorti, and Contaldo. "Postprandial Thermogenesis in Lean and Obese Subjects after Meals Supplemented with Medium-Chain and Long-Chain Triglycerides." *American Journal of Clinical Nutrition* (May 1991). http://www.ncbi.nlm.nih.gov/pubmed/2021124.

Seaton, Welle, Warenko, and Campbell. "Thermic Effect of Medium-Chain and Long-Chain Triglycerides in Man." *American Journal of Clinical Nutrition* (November 1986). http://www.ncbi.nlm.nih.gov/pubmed/3532757.

Simopoulos. "The Importance of the Ratio of Omega-6/Omega-3 Essential Fatty Acids." 2002. http://www.ncbi.nlm.nih.gov/pubmed/12442909.

van Wymelbeke, Himaya, Louis-Sylvestre, and Fantino. "Influence of Medium-Chain and Long-Chain Triacylglycerols on the Control of Food Intake in Men." *American Journal of Clinical Nutrition* (August 1998). http://www.ncbi.nlm.nih.gov/pubmed/9701177.

Wang and Tong. "The Key Enzyme of Cholesterol Synthesis Pathway: HMG-COA Reductase and Disease." *Sheng Li Ke Xue Jin Zhan* 30, no. 1 (January 1999): 5–9.

Willett, Sacks, and Stampfer. "Dietary Fat and Heart Disease Study Is Seriously Misleading." *Nutrition Source*, (March 19, 2014).

http://www.hsph.harvard.edu/nutritionsource/2014/03/19/
dietary-fat-and-heart-disease-study-is-seriously-misleading/.

Zheng, Xu, Li, Liu, Hui, and Huang. "Green Tea Intake Lowers
Fasting Serum Total and LDL Cholesterol in Adults: A Meta-
Analysis of 14 Randomized Controlled Trials." *American Journal
of Clinical Nutrition* (August 2011). http://www.ncbi.nlm.nih.gov/
pubmed/21715508.

Studies; Digestion

Ali, Choe, Awab, Wagener, and Orr. "Sleep, Immunity and Inflammation
in Gastrointestinal Disorders." *World Journal of Gastroenterology*
(December 28, 2013). http://www.ncbi.nlm.nih.gov/pmc/articles/
PMC3882397/.

Dantas and Aben-Athar. "Aspects of Sleep Effects on the Digestive
Tract." *Arquivos de gastroenterologia* 1 (January–March 2002): 55–9.
http://www.ncbi.nlm.nih.gov/pubmed/12184167.

Fass. "Sleep and Gastroesophageal Reflux Disease (GERD)." *Digestive
Health Matters* 21, no. 2 (June 2012). http://www.aboutgerd.org/
site/symptoms/sleep-and-gerd.

Jenkins, Wolever, Leeds, Gassull, Haisman, Dilawari, Goff, Metz, and
Alberti. "Dietary Fibres, Fibre Analogues, and Glucose Tolerance:
Importance of Viscosity." *British Medical Journal* (1978). http://
www.bmj.com/content/1/6124/1392.

Jung, Choung, and Talley. "Gastroesophageal Reflux Disease and
Sleep Disorders: Evidence for a Causal Link and Therapeutic
Implications." *Journal of Neurogastroenterology and Motility* (January
2010). http://www.ncbi.nlm.nih.gov/pmc/articles/PMC2879818/.

Muller, Fullwood, Hawkins, and Cowley. "The Integrated Response of the Cardiovascular System to Food." *Digestion* (1992). http://www. ncbi.nlm.nih.gov/pubmed/1459353

Studies; Exercise

Body, Bergmann, Boonen, Boutsen, Bruyere, Devogelaer, Goemaere, et al. "Non-Pharmacological Management of Osteoporosis: A Consensus of the Belgian Bone Club." *Osteoporosis International* (November 2011). http://www.ncbi.nlm.nih.gov/pmc/articles/ PMC3186889/.

Bonaiuti, Shea, Iovine, Negrini, Robinson, Kemper, Wells, Tugwell, and Cranney. "Exercise for Preventing and Treating Osteoporosis in Postmenopausal Women." *Cochrane Database of Systematic Reviews* (2002). http://www.ncbi.nlm.nih.gov/pubmed/12137611.

Buman and King. "Exercise as a Treatment to Enhance Sleep." *American Journal of Lifestyle Medicine* (November/December 2010). http://ajl. sagepub.com/content/4/6/500.abstract.

Erickson, Voss, Prakash, Basak, Szabo, Chaddock, Kim, et al. "Exercise Training Increases Size of Hippocampus and Improves Memory." Proceedings of the National Academy of Sciences USA (February 15, 2011). http://www.ncbi.nlm.nih.gov/pmc/articles/PMC3041121/.

Hamer, Stamatakis, and Steptoe. "Dose-Response Relationship between Physical Activity and Mental Health: The Scottish Health Survey." *British Journal of Sports Medicine* (2009). http://www.ncbi. nlm.nih.gov/pubmed/18403415.

Harber and Sutton. "Endorphins and Exercise." *Sports Medicine* (1984). http://www.ncbi.nlm.nih.gov/pubmed/6091217.

Hayes, Bickerstaff, and Baker. "Interactions of Cortisol, Testosterone, and Resistance Training: Influence of Circadian Rhythms." *Chronobiology International* (June 2010). http://www.ncbi.nlm.nih.gov/pubmed/20560706.

Healy, Dunstan, Salmon, Cerin, Shaw, Zimmet, et al. "Breaks in Sedentary Time: Beneficial Associations with Metabolic Risk." *Diabetes Care* (2008). http://www.ncbi.nlm.nih.gov/pubmed/18252901.

Hertzog, Kramer, Wilson, and Lindenberger. "Enrichment Effects on Adult Cognitive Development: Can the Functional Capacity of Older Adults Be Preserved and Enhanced?" *Psychological Science in the Public Interest* (2008). http://www.psychologicalscience.org/journals/pspi/pdf/PSPI_9_1%20main_text.pdf.

Owen, Bauman, and Brown. "Too Much Sitting: A Novel and Important Predictor of Chronic Disease Risk?" *Medicine and Science in Sports and Exercise* (2009). http://www.ncbi.nlm.nih.gov/pubmed/19346988.

Patel, Bernstein, Deka, Feigelson, Campbell, Gapstur, et al. "Leisure Time Spent Sitting in Relation to Total Mortality in a Prospective Cohort of US Adults." *American Journal of Epidemiology* (2010). http://www.ncbi.nlm.nih.gov/pubmed/20650954.

Pedersen and Febbraio. "Muscles, Exercise and Obesity: Skeletal Muscle as a Secretory Organ." *Nature Reviews Endocrinology* (2012). http://www.nature.com/nrendo/journal/v8/n8/full/nrendo.2012.49.html

Sparling, Giuffrida, Piomelli, Rosskopf, and Dietrich. "Exercise Activates the Endocannabinoid System." *Neuroreport* 14, no. 17 (December 2003): 2209–211. http://journals.lww.com/neuroreport/Abstract/2003/12020/Exercise_activates_the_endocannabinoid_system.15.aspx.

Strawbridge, Deleger, Roberts, and Kaplan. "Physical Activity Reduces the Risk of Subsequent Depression for Older Adults." *American Journal of Epidemiology* 1 (2002). http://www.ncbi.nlm.nih.gov/pubmed/12181102.

Van Proeyen, Szlufcik, Nielens, Pelgrim, Deldicque, Hesselink, van Veldhoven, and Hespel. "Training in the Fasted State Improves Glucose Tolerance during Fat-Rich Diet." *Journal of Physiology* (2010). http://www.ncbi.nlm.nih.gov/pubmed/20837645.

Van Proeyen, Szlufcik, Nielens, Ramaekers, and Hespel. "Beneficial Metabolic Adaptations Due to Endurance Exercise Training in the Fasted State." *Journal of Applied Physiology* (2011). http://www.ncbi.nlm.nih.gov/nlmcatalog?term=%22J+Appl+Physiol+(1985)%22[Title+Abbreviation.

Youngstedt. "Effects of Exercise on Sleep." *Clinics in Sports Medicine* (2005). http://www.ncbi.nlm.nih.gov/pubmed/15892929.

Studies; Fat Cells

Grégoire, Genart, Hauser, and Remacle. "Glucocorticoids Induce a Drastic Inhibition of Proliferation and Stimulate Differentiation of Adult Rat Fat Cell Precursors." *Experimental Cell Research* (October 1991). http://www.ncbi.nlm.nih.gov/pubmed/1893938.

Hauner, Schmid, and Pfeiffer. "Glucocorticoids and Insulin Promote the Differentiation of Human Adipocyte Precursor Cells into Fat Cells." (April 1987). http://www.ncbi.nlm.nih.gov/pubmed/3546356.

Jeyakumar, Vajreswari, Sesikeran, and Giridharan. "Vitamin A Supplementation Induces Adipose Tissue Loss through Apoptosis in Lean but Not in Obese Rats of the WNIN/OB Strain." *Journal of Molecular Endocrinology* (October 1, 2005). http://jme.endocrinology-journals.org/content/35/2/391.full.

Studies; Hormones; Cortisol

Chan and Debono. "Replication of Cortisol Circadian Rhythm: New Advances in Hydrocortisone Replacement Therapy." *Therapeutic Advances in Endocrinology and Metabolism* (June 2010). http://www.ncbi.nlm.nih.gov/pmc/articles/PMC3475279/.

Hayes, Bickerstaff, and Baker. "Interactions of Cortisol, Testosterone, and Resistance Training: Influence of Circadian Rhythms." *Chronobiology International* (June 2010). http://www.ncbi.nlm.nih.gov/pubmed/20560706.

Studies; Hormones; Ghrelin

Blom, Lluch, Stafleu, Vinoy, Holst, Schaafsma, and Hendriks. "Effect of a High-Protein Breakfast on the Postprandial Ghrelin Response." *American Journal of Clinical Nutrition* (2006). http://ajcn.nutrition.org/content/83/2/211.full.

Callahan, Cummings, Pepe, Breen, Matthys, and Weigle. "Postprandial Suppression of Plasma Ghrelin Level Is Proportional to Ingested Caloric Load but Does Not Predict Intermeal Interval in Humans." *Journal of Clinical Endocrinology and Metabolism* (March 2004). http://www.ncbi.nlm.nih.gov/pubmed/15001628.

Chen, Asakawa, Fujimiya, Lee, and Inui. "Ghrelin Gene Products and the Regulation of Food Intake and Gut Motility." *Pharmacological Reviews* (December 2009). http://pharmrev.aspetjournals.org/content/61/4/430.full#ref-91.

Kim, Yoon, Jang, Park, Shin, Park, Ryu, et al. "The Mitogenic and Antiapoptotic Actions of Ghrelin in 3t3-L1 Adipocytes." *Molecular Endocrinology* (September 2004). http://www.ncbi.nlm.nih.gov/pubmed/15178745.

Koliaki, Kokkinos, Tentolouris, and Katsilambros. "The Effect of Ingested Macronutrients on Postprandial Ghrelin Response: A Critical Review of Existing Literature Data." *International Journal of Peptides* (2010). http://www.hindawi.com/journals/ijpep/2010/710852/.

Schmid, Hallschmid, Jauch-Chara, Born, and Schultes. "A Single Night of Sleep Deprivation Increases Ghrelin Levels and Feelings of Hunger in Normal-Weight Healthy Men." *Journal of Sleep Research* (September 2008). http://www.ncbi.nlm.nih.gov/pubmed/18564298.

Sugino, Yamaura, Yamagishi, Ogura, Hayashi, Kurose, Kojima, et al. "A Transient Surge of Ghrelin Secretion before Feeding Is Modified by Different Feeding Regimens in Sheep." *Biochemical and Biophysical Research Communications* (November 15, 2002). http://www.ncbi.nlm.nih.gov/pubmed/12419323.

Studies; Hormones; Insulin

Claessens, Saris, and van Baak. "Glucagon and Insulin Responses after Ingestion of Different Amounts of Intact and Hydrolysed Proteins." *British Journal of Nutrition* (2008). http://www.ncbi.nlm.nih.gov/pubmed/18167171.

Duckworth, Bennett, and Hamel. "Insulin Degradation: Progress and Potential." *Endocrine Reviews* (July 1, 2013). http://press.endocrine.org/doi/full/10.1210/edrv.19.5.0349.

Jakubowicz, Wainstein, Bar-Dayan, Rabinovitz, and Froy. "Differential Morning vs. Evening Insulin and Glucagon-Like Peptide-1 (GLP-1) Responses after Identical Meal in Type 2 Diabetic Subjects." *Endocrine Society* (June 2014). http://press. endocrine.org/doi/abs/10.1210/endo-meetings.2014.DGM.16. SUN-1058.

Jensen, Rustad, Kolnes, and Lai. "Role of Skeletal Muscle Glycogen Breakdown for Regulation of Insulin Sensitivity by Exercise." *Frontiers in Physiology* 2 (2011): 112. http://www.ncbi.nlm.nih.gov/ pmc/articles/PMC3248697/.

Ji, Guan, Frank, and Messina. "Insulin Inhibits Growth Hormone Signaling via the Growth Hormone Receptor/JAK2/STAT5B Pathway." *Journal of Biological Chemistry* (May 7, 1999). http://www. jbc.org/content/274/19/13434.full.

Lanzi, Luzi, Caumo, Andreotti, Manzoni, Malighetti, Sereni, and Pontiroli. "Elevated Insulin Levels Contribute to the Reduced Growth Hormone (GH) Response to GH-Releasing Hormone in Obese Subjects." *Metabolism* (1999). http://www.ncbi.nlm.nih.gov/ pubmed/10484056.

McClenaghan, Barnett, O'Harte, and Flatt. "Mechanisms of Amino Acid-Induced Insulin Secretion from the Glucose-Responsive Brin-Bd11 Pancreatic B-Cell Line." *Journal of Endocrinology* (December 1996). http://www.ncbi.nlm.nih.gov/pubmed/8994380.

Ness and Chambers. "Feedback and Hormonal Regulation of Hepatic 3-Hydroxy-3-Methylglutaryl Coenzyme A Reductase: The Concept of Cholesterol Buffering Capacity." *Proceedings of the Society for Experimental Biology and Medicine* 224, no. 1 (May 2000): 8–19. http://www.ncbi.nlm.nih.gov/pubmed/10782041.

Nuttall, Mooradian, Gannon, Billington, and Krezowski. "Effect of Protein Ingestion on the Glucose and Insulin Response to a Standardized Oral Glucose Load." *Diabetes Care* (1984). http://care.diabetesjournals.org/content/7/5/465.

Steinberger and Daniels. "Obesity, Insulin Resistance, Diabetes, and Cardiovascular Risk in Children." *Circulation Journal* (2003). http://circ.ahajournals.org/content/107/10/1448.long.

Valera Mora, Scarfone, Calvani, Greco, and Mingrone. "Insulin Clearance in Obesity." *Journal of the American College of Nutrition* (December 2003). http://www.ncbi.nlm.nih.gov/pubmed/14684753.

Van Loon, Saris, Verhagen, and Wagenmakers. "Plasma Insulin Responses after Ingestion of Different Amino Acid or Protein Mixtures with Carbohydrate." *American Journal of Clinical Nutrition* (2000). http://ajcn.nutrition.org/content/72/1/96.long.

Van Loon, Kruijshoop, Menheere, Wagenmakers, Saris, and Keizer. "Amino Acid Ingestion Strongly Enhances Insulin Secretion in Patients with Long-Term Type 2 Diabetes." *Diabetes Care* (2003). http://care.diabetesjournals.org/content/26/3/625.full.

Zorzano, Balon, Goodman, and Ruderman. "Glycogen Depletion and Increased Insulin Sensitivity and Responsiveness in Muscle after Exercise." *American Journal of Physiology* 1 (December 25, 1986). 664–69. http://www.ncbi.nlm.nih.gov/pubmed/3538900.

Studies; Hormones; Leptin

Farooqi, Matarese, Lord, Keogh, Lawrence, Agwu, Sanna, et al. "Beneficial Effects of Leptin on Obesity: T Cell Hyporesponsiveness, and Neuroendocrine/Metabolic Dysfunction of Human Congenital

Leptin Deficiency." *Journal of Clinical Investigation* (October 15, 2002). http://www.ncbi.nlm.nih.gov/pmc/articles/PMC150795/.

Jéquier and Tappy. "Regulation of Body Weight in Humans." *Physiological Reviews* 79, no. 2 (April 1999). http://physrev.physiology.org/content/79/2/451.

Sarmiento, Benson, Kaufman, Ross, Scully, and DiPalma. "Morphologic and Molecular Changes Induced by Recombinant Human Leptin in the White and Brown Adipose Tissues of C57bl/6 Mice." *Laboratory Investigation* (September 1997). http://www.ncbi.nlm.nih.gov/pubmed/9314948.

Wang, Pan, Lee, Kakuma, Zhou, and Unger. "The Role of Leptin Resistance in the Lipid Abnormalities of Aging." *FASEB Journal* (January 2001). http://www.ncbi.nlm.nih.gov/pubmed/11149898.

Studies; Hormones; Growth Hormone

"Growth Hormone, Athletic Performance, and Aging." *Harvard Health Publications* (May, 2010). http://www.health.harvard.edu/newsletters/Harvard_Mens_Health_Watch/2010/May/growth-hormone-athletic-performance-and-aging.

Imura, Kato, Ikeda, Morimoto, and Yawata. "Effect of Adrenergic-Blocking or -Stimulating Agents on Plasma Growth Hormone, Immunoreactive Insulin, and Blood Free Fatty Acid Levels in Man." *Journal of Clinical Investigation* 50, no. 5 (May 1971). http://www.jci.org/articles/view/106578.

Ji, Guan, Frank, and Messina. "Insulin Inhibits Growth Hormone Signaling via the Growth Hormone Receptor/JAK2/STAT5B

Pathway." *Journal of Biological Chemistry* (May 7, 1999). http://www.jbc.org/content/274/19/13434.full.

Lanzi, Luzi, Caumo, Andreotti, Manzoni, Malighetti, Sereni, and Pontiroli. "Elevated Insulin Levels Contribute to the Reduced Growth Hormone (GH) Response to GH-Releasing Hormone in Obese Subjects." *Metabolism* (1999). http://www.ncbi.nlm.nih.gov/pubmed/10484056.

Reed, Merriam, and Kargi. "Adult Growth Hormone Deficiency: Benefits, Side Effects, and Risks of Growth Hormone Replacement." *Frontiers in Endocrinology* (2013). http://www.ncbi.nlm.nih.gov/pmc/articles/PMC3671347/.

Sattler, "Growth Hormone in the Aging Male." *Clinical Endocrinological Metabolism* (August 2013). http://*www*.ncbi.nlm.nih.gov/pmc/articles/PMC3940699/.

Takahashi, *Kipnis*, and Daughaday. "Growth Hormone Secretion during Sleep." *Journal of Clinical Investigation* 47, no. 9 (September 1968): 2079–90. http://www.ncbi.nlm.nih.gov/pmc/articles/PMC297368/pdf/jcinvest00244-0147.pdf.

Van Cauter and Plat, "Physiology of Growth Hormone Secretion during Sleep." *Journal of Pediatrics* (1996). http://www.ncbi.nlm.nih.gov/pubmed/8627466.

Studies; Other

Adam and Mercer. "Appetite Regulation and Seasonality: Implications for Obesity." *Proceedings of the Nutrition Society* (2004). http://journals.cambridge.org/download.php?file=%2FPNS%2FPNS63_03

%2FS0029665104000564a.pdf&code=6a678e2eed7163170244640 216120c97.

Alirezaei, Kemball, Flynn, Wood, Whitton, and Kiosses. "Short-Term Fasting Induces Profound Neuronal Autophagy." *Autophagy (August 2010)*. http://www.ncbi.nlm.nih.gov/pubmed/20534972.

Bergamini, Cavallini, Donati, and Gori. "The Role of Autophagy in Aging: Its Essential Part in the Anti-Aging Mechanism of Caloric Restriction." *Annals of the New York Academy of Sciences* (2007). http://www.ncbi.nlm.nih.gov/pubmed/17934054.

Bergström, Fürst, Norée, and Vinnars. "Intracellular Free Amino Acid Concentration in Human Muscle Tissue." *Journal of Applied Physiology* (1974). http://jap.physiology.org/content/36/6/693.full. pdf.

Di Stasi, MacLeod, Winters, and Binder-Macleod., "Effects of Statins on Skeletal Muscle: A Perspective for Physical Therapists." *Journal of American Physical Therapy Association* (October 2010). http://www. ncbi.nlm.nih.gov/pmc/articles/PMC2949584/.

Fenton, Lyon, Eliasziw, Tough, and Hanley. "Meta-Analysis of the Effect of the Acid-Ash Hypothesis of Osteoporosis on Calcium Balance." *Journal of Bone and Mineral Research* (2009). http://www. ncbi.nlm.nih.gov/pubmed/19419322.

Gangwisch, Heymsfield, Boden-Albala, Buijs, Kreier, Pickering, et al. "Short Sleep Duration as a Risk Factor for Hypertension: Analyses of the First National Health and Nutrition Examination Survey." *Hypertension* (May 2006). http://www.ncbi.nlm.nih.gov/ pubmed/16585410.

Grandner, Patel, Gehrman, Perlis, and Pack. "Problems Associated with Short Sleep: Bridging the Gap between Laboratory and Epidemiological Studies." *Sleep Medicine Reviews* (August 2010). http://www.ncbi.nlm.nih.gov/pmc/articles/PMC2888649/.

Kennedy, Martinez, Schmidt, Mandrup, LaPoint, and McIntosh. "Antiobesity Mechanisms of Action of Conjugated Linoleic Acid." *Journal of Nutritional Biochemistry*, (December 2009). http://www.ncbi.nlm.nih.gov/pmc/articles/PMC2826589/.

Kim and Lemasters. "Mitochondrial Degradation by Autophagy (Mitophagy) in GFP-LC3 Transgenic Hepatocytes during Nutrient Deprivation." *American Journal of Physiology, Cell Physiology* (February 2011). http://www.ncbi.nlm.nih.gov/pubmed/21106691.

Kreitzman, Coxon, and Szaz. "Glycogen Storage: Illusions of Easy Weight Loss, Excessive Weight Regain, and Distortions in Estimates of Body Composition." *American Journal of Clinical Nutrition* (July 1992). http://ajcn.nutrition.org/content/56/1/292S.long.

Masiero, Agatea, Mammucari, Blaauw, Loro, Komatsu, Metzger, Reggiani, Schiaffino, and Sandri. "Autophagy Is Required to Maintain Muscle Mass." *Cell Metabolism* (2009). http://www.ncbi.nlm.nih.gov/pubmed/19945408.

Olsson and Saltin. "Variation in Total Body Water with Muscle Glycogen Changes in Man." *Acta physiologica Scandinavica* (September 1970). http://onlinelibrary.wiley.com/doi/10.1111/j.1748-1716.1970.tb04764.x/abstract;jsessionid=EFED180858B56C048802245B3A0F1E80.f02t04.

Ray, Seshasai, Erqou, Sever, Jukema, Ford, and Sattar. "Statins and All-Cause Mortality in High-Risk Primary Prevention: A Meta-Analysis

Maimonides & Metabolism

of 11 Randomized Controlled Trials Involving 65,229 Participants." *Archives of Internal Medicine* (June 28, 2010). http://www.ncbi.nlm. nih.gov/pubmed/20585067.

Schwenke. "Seasonal Fluctuation in Weight is Not Associated with Weight Gain." *Circulation* (2010). http://circ.ahajournals.org/cgi/content/meeting_abstract/122/21_MeetingAbstracts/A21291.

Sherman, Plyley, Sharp, van Handel, McAllister, W. J. Fink, and D. L. Costill. "Muscle Glycogen Storage and Its Relationship with Water." *International Journal of Sports Medicine* (February 1982). http://www.ncbi.nlm.nih.gov/pubmed/7068293.

Sukhija, Prayaga, Marashdeh, Bursac, Kakar, Bansal, Sachdeva, Kesan, and Mehta. "Effect of Statins on Fasting Plasma Glucose in Diabetic and Nondiabetic Patients." *Journal of Investigative Medicine* (March 2009). http://www.ncbi.nlm.nih.gov/pubmed/19188844?dopt=Abstract.

Van Leeuwen, Lehto, Karisola, Lindholm, Luukkonen, Sallinen, et al. "Sleep Restriction Increases the Risk of Developing Cardiovascular Diseases by Augmenting Pro-Inflammatory Responses through Il-17 and CRP." *PLoS ONE* (2009). http://www.ncbi.nlm.nih.gov/pmc/articles/PMC2643002/.

Websites

American Heart Association, http://www.heart.org/idc/groups/heart-public/@wcm/@hcm/documents/downloadable/ucm_300322.pdf.

American Diabetes Association, "Glycemic Index and Diabetes." last modified May 14, 2004, http://www.diabetes.org/food-and-fitness/food/what-can-i-eat/understanding-carbohydrates/glycemic-index-and-diabetes.html.

316

Bazian. "Saturated Fats and Heart Disease Link 'Unproven,'" *Behind the Headlines: Health News from NHS Choices* (March 18, 2014), http://www.nhs.uk/news/2014/03march/pages/saturated-fats-and-heart-disease-link-unproven.aspx.

Clinical Advisor. "Vitamin D Aids Weight Loss in Obese, Overweight Patients." http://www.clinicaladvisor.com/web-exclusives/vitamin-d-weight-loss-obese-overweight-deficiency/article/413772/

National Heart Lung and Blood Institute of the US Department of Health and Human Services, National Institutes of Health. http://www.nhlbi.nih.gov/health/health-topics/topics/ms/.

National Lipids Association. http://www.lipidjournal.com/pb/assets/raw/Health%20Advance/journals/jacl/NLA_Recommendations_manuscript.pdf.

Red Orbit Staff and Wire Reports. "Trans Fats from Ruminant Animals May Be Beneficial." *Red Orbit* (September 8, 2011). http://www.redorbit.com/news/health/2608879/trans-fats-from-ruminant-animals-may-be-beneficial/.

US Department of Agriculture, US Department of Health and Human Services www.dietaryguidelines.gov.